SELENIUM

The amazing discoveries behind this vital substance and how we can benefit from its preventive and healing properties.

SELENIUM

The Essential Trace Element You Might Not Be Getting Enough Of

by

ALAN LEWIS

THORSONS PUBLISHERS LIMITED
Wellingborough, Northamptonshire

First published 1982
Revised and expanded 1983

British Library Cataloguing in Publication Data

Lewis, Alan,
    Selenium.—Rev. & expanded ed.
    1. Selenium in human nutrition
    613.2'8   TX553.S4

    ISBN 0-7225-0917-0

Printed and bound in Great Britain

CONTENTS

		Page
Foreword by Dr Dick Richards		7
Introduction		9
Chapter		
1.	Trace Elements – 'The Poor Relations'	13
2.	Astounding Facts and Figures	19
3.	A Victory Against Arthritis	23
4.	The Success Stories	33
5.	Can You Really Stay Younger Longer?	37
6.	Fighting Cancer Naturally	49
7.	Towards a Healthier Heart	61
8.	Vitamin E and Selenium – a Great Double Act	68
9.	Selenium in Our Food	73
10	What of the Future?	81
11	'Thank You for Helping Me'	91
	Index	95

When this book on selenium was first printed the research into selenium all over the world was growing almost month by month. The potential of this trace element has since then awakened fresh medical interest in almost every country in the world from Japan to New Zealand and from Britain to the United States.

International symposiums are now held somewhere in the world every year to update and reveal new evidence.

In an expanded version of this book I have looked in detail at the way selenium has come to the fore in Britain as a success story in the cure of arthritis and rheumatism. It also looks at fresh studies into cancer research and that particular connection with selenium.

I would like to thank the British Arthritic Association and *Here's Health* magazine for help in the chapters relating to selenium and arthritis.

FOREWORD

Only a few short years ago no-one but a handful of scientists would have heard of selenium. Even they had little idea of its importance... yet it was and is vital to the healthy lives of everyone.

Apart from occasional academic papers in learned publications, such material as appeared for the general public to read was either confused and inadequate or frankly prejudiced. Nevertheless, throughout the world, pioneers were gradually noticing, trying, and being impressed by the success of selenium dietary supplements. A few of these were qualified doctors and experts. Most were naturopaths, clinical ecologists and nutritionists.

Their approach was that if an idea worked and was safe, then it should be used despite the lack of published evidence. Then, given time, research could catch up and prove them right. It was in this way that vitamin A and the correct diet were in use as the powerful cancer preventers they are, long before orthodox physicians realized what they and their patients were missing.

So it was with selenium, too. The evidence is now

overwhelming, both clinical and documentary, that selenium is of preventive and therapeutic value in arthritis, heart disease and cancer. And new discoveries are on the way.

Alan Lewis's book is full of data and logic. His presentation of the case for selenium is flawless. Any reader will discover what took me half a professional lifetime; that selenium should be recommended and taken . . . always. There is no longer any reason to hold back.

DR DICK RICHARDS
Harley Street
London

INTRODUCTION

Ted Greene is a quite remarkable man. But then so is Bill Sutton. The same might also be said of Billy Collins and his wife Amy. In fact, you do not have to wander far from this rather special group of people to find a whole lot more extraordinary human beings. And what they share is two important things. The first is where they live; the second is their considerable age. Ted, for example, is 91. Billy Collins is 96, his wife Amy is 91. Bill Sutton is a relative youngster at 76. The part of England they share as their home is a few square miles of the North Norfolk coast which is now being acknowledged as one of the most extraordinary corners of the United Kingdom. Within this tiny area, the people live longer than anywhere else in Britain, and this is not just an assumption, it's a statistical fact.

The area boasts four active centenarians. There is also a choir where the average age is 73; a gardening association specially formed for the elderly, average age 71; a Darby and Joan club, average age 74.

A lot of trouble has arisen and feelings have been hurt

because the local over 70's club has more members than it can cope with – and a waiting list. A look round the local cemeteries in the area shows that it is not a recent thing. The life expectancy has, for several generations, been very high.

Longevity in the Andes

Studies into great age, whether it be in the remote highlands of the Andes, where there have existed communities of people who may live for 140 years, or in a more remote area of the Indian continent, have produced a formula. It seems that, quite simply, the answer lies in the soil. Almost all of the detailed studies have found that centenarians are closely involved with the land, and that the bulk of their food is grown locally. It has now been statistically established that people working in agriculture live the longest. They are closely followed by clergymen and then come naturalists. These same three groups of people also have the lowest incidence of cancer. Is it possible that the connection may be that, through the years, they were poor people who could not afford rich food? Simple, plain food, often home-grown fruit and vegetables was not just a choice – it was an economic necessity.

At the other end of the scale, groups who tend to die early include film stars, lawyers and journalists – jobs which are normally associated with stress and tension and linked with city life. It is also these three groups which suffer most from ulcers and stomach cancer.

Diet and the Ageing Process

The subject of ageing and long life has always fascinated people. Scientists have naturally been keen to know more about the ageing process. What are the factors? Is there any formula which is more likely to work or make sense than others? Is diet important? Is old age linked to hereditary factors?

Slowly a pattern has been built up. And it is a pattern which reveals that old age is most frequent where the diet is frugal and low in calories; the age factor is also closely linked to the type of soil, from which most of the food is taken.

This takes us back to North Norfolk and a thriving community where the days of poverty may be a thing of the past, but where the other parts of the formula still remain. It is a community which relies very heavily on allotments and vegetable gardens to provide home-grown fruit and vegetables for an area which has an above average number of retired people. It is the connection with the soil that is the key factor both in this case and in all the important discoveries made in more remote areas; the trace elements that exist in the soil are of vital importance. The centenarians all lived surrounded by high mountains. Trace elements were deposited in the valleys where the soil was rich in minerals and they, in turn, were passed on through the food grown there.

One of the most vital of the 20 or so trace elements that the body needs is selenium. It occurs naturally in the soil and exists in small amounts in foods such as wholegrain wheat, brewer's yeast, sesame seeds, garlic, mushrooms and fish or shell-fish.

Trace elements have been one of the most important and exciting fields of discovery in recent years. The interplay of various elements, which the body needs in such small amounts, is now the subject of intense research work at centres throughout the world. But what is known already is that selenium makes things happen in the body to such an extent that it helps prevent high blood pressure; it can also be an effective therapy for angina and is vital for healthy heart muscles.

We all need selenium, and although it occurs naturally in the soil, the vast majority of us are not getting enough of this particular element – even if we eat the right sort of selenium-rich foods. In fact, there is only one area of the U.K. where the diet provides the necessary amount of selenium. You have guessed it – those few miles of the North Norfolk coast where it has now been proved that people live longer than anywhere else on these islands.

And why is this? The people do not have a particularly easy life. They do, however, live away from stress and many of them have lived in the area all their lives and grown fruit and vegetables in their gardens. Plain food is still the order of the day.

What this book sets out to do is try and find the answer. It looks into the belief that what was, until very recently, a little known trace element could hold some very considerable secrets regarding our health and well-being. On the way, this book tries to unravel some of the mysteries of why some people live longer and much more active lives than others; it is partly a detective story, trying to unscramble conflicting evidence and theories. Another part of it is a scientific story, looking into the science of trace elements, their importance for the body and the world-wide studies into every aspect of selenium.

One thing is certain. The story of selenium is here to stay and in the years ahead it may be seen as one of the most vital breakthroughs ever seen in man's understanding of his own body and how it can best be cared for.

1.

TRACE ELEMENTS –
'THE POOR RELATIONS'

More than 5,000 trainee nurses recently took part in a survey to find out how much they knew about nutrition. Nine out of ten cound not answer the following question: 'What are trace elements? Why are they so important to the body?' The nurses, who took the test after two years of their training, knew all they needed to know about vitamins and vitamin deficiency, they were not quite so well up on minerals, and knew almost nothing about trace elements. It may not necessarily be their fault, nor indeed are they the only ones to suffer from such a gap in their knowledge. For while more people than ever are conscious of the importance of vitamins, how many are aware that trace elements and trace minerals are just as vital for health?

The message that ill health is not just a question of luck, but is directly linked to what we eat and our general lifestyles, is beginning to be appreciated as never before. There is a move towards eating more fresh vegetables, fruit, salads, wholemeal bread and flour, towards fitness and exercise. At the same time, there is concern about eating processed foods, as well as the dangers of too many fats and the harmful effects of sugar in the diet. All this is part of a growing awareness of the fact that eating habits have been going wrong and that by putting them right, we can promote good health.

So, quite naturally, the role of vitamins is high-lighted. Everyone is more 'vitamin conscious'. Food manufacturers display 'Added Vitamins' and 'Extra Vitamins' on their packaging of everything from breakfast cereals to fruit juices in an attempt to take advantage of that consciousness. But is the same true about minerals? And is the same true about trace minerals and trace elements? Nutritionists now refuse to distinguish between the degrees of importance to our diet of vitamins, minerals and trace elements. They are all equally vital.

The Importance of Minerals in the Diet
It was not very long ago that the full importance of minerals was realized. Very little was known about the precise role they had to play and many people's knowledge of minerals may well have been summed up in two sentences: 'If you are anaemic you need iron', and 'Calcium is good for your teeth and your bones'. Thankfully, all that has changed. We now know so much more about the role and function of magnesium, zinc, phosphorus, potassium, chromium, manganese and so on. We know more about what happens when we do not get enough of them, which foods contain which minerals and how and when you should increase the mineral value of your diet.

Research at all levels in centres throughout the world has, in the past twenty years, shown that a lack of minerals in the daily diet can be just as serious as a lack of vitamins. Yet the public's knowledge of them falls far short of the strides made to make housewives and parents more vitamin conscious.

Within the whole study of minerals, one important factor has repeatedly emerged; the importance of some minerals which the body needs in very, very small quantities

- even one millionth of a gram. These have become known as trace elements. Deficiency of these trace elements has caused illness, just as serious as those caused by deficiencies of some vitamins and minerals which the body needs in much greater amounts.

The study of trace elements is a new science compared with the steps taken fifty or so years ago to isolate and identify vitamins from food sources. Vitamins such as A, B-complex, C, D, E, and K were all isolated and named between 1926 and 1948. Each vitamin has, in its time, been the subject of a steadily increasing volume of research and our knowledge of them is sophisticated and detailed. So if the first half of this century very much belongs to the discovery of vitamins, then we must allocate much of the second half to the growth in what we know about minerals. Until this century, only iodine and iron had undergone sufficient laboratory tests to reveal that they could combat diseases which stemmed from poor diets; and it is only since 1950 that methods for detecting and measuring trace elements have been developed enough for us to realize fully how vital they are.

Mineral Sources and Deficiencies

The principal source of minerals is the soil and whereas vitamins are brought together or synthesized by plants and animals, minerals must come from outside. And that goes some way towards explaining why essential elements are still being recognized and the depth and range of knowledge will increase in the years to come.

Minerals cannot be made by the body and so we depend on our food and water intake to provide the amount we need. Therefore, our source of minerals must be the soil; and the way plants take minerals up from the soil is the essence of the whole equation which governs the quantity and quality of the amount of these essential minerals which eventually find their way into our diets and which maintain our health. Our bodies need many more minerals for good health than plants do for growth. Plants need only fifteen or so nutrients; our bodies need over fifty. The whole equation of the mineral content of the soil in which our food grows, right through to the way our body absorbs or fails to absorb the nutrients, is a complex one.

To start with, the richness of the soil varies enormously – not only in the quantity of the minor minerals and trace elements, but even in the major nutrients such as nitrogen, phosphorus and potassium, which are commonly associated with the soil any gardener would be proud of. And as the richness varies, so deficiencies in the soil can be noted. Where there are deficiencies, medical research can translate them into a direct effect on the health and well-being of the people who live in those areas.

Large portions of the Mid-western States of America are deficient in iodine, a mineral known to be an essential part of some hormones. An iodine deficiency leads to the whole action of the body slowing down and an enlargement of the thyroid gland or goitre. Those same areas of the United States, identified as being poor in iodine content are infamous for the number of goitre cases recorded there. Inland limestone areas are normally the most deficient and, in the United Kingdom, Derbyshire is one such area.

The incidence of cancer, leukaemia and heart disease can all be related to areas which show deficiencies in different minerals. Time and again, the basic calculations of the number of people suffering from these diseases, related to deficiencies in the soil in areas where they occur, show there is a firm connection. It becomes a fact of life that some people are more likely to catch major diseases and become seriously ill because of where they live. For instance, in some areas of France and Belgium the low magnesium content of the soil is associated with an above average number of people suffering from cancer. International studies in the Middle East have directly linked a low intake of zinc with the high number of dwarfs found there. In addition, areas of Asia, the Eastern United States and Switzerland, where there is a chromium deficiency, are known to be areas where heart-related diseases are high. As the story of this book develops, we shall see the way in which selenium, perhaps more than any other mineral, plays a vital health-giving role – just by being present in the soil.

It is still possible to underestimate the value of minerals, as we have seen, since they seem destined never to be quite as fashionable as their vitamin cousins. But although it is true to say that far less is known about the way minerals work in the body than vitamins, it is equally true that many deficiencies have been isolated and we do know, for instance, that: calcium is vital for bone growth and deficiency can cause kidney failure, spasms and loss of muscle power; lack of chromium upsets the body's ability to turn food into energy and is linked with heart troubles; copper deficiency can lead to general weakness, hair and heart problems; iodine deficiency can result in enlarged thyroid glands; iron is vital for the health of the blood and lack of this mineral can bring tiredness and a lower resistance to illness; magnesium has a direct effect on the health of the heart; manganese is essential for growth, reproduction and skeleton development; zinc deficiency slows down the body's ability to heal wounds and has been linked with decreasing a child's growth rate.

It is a list which shows how we are learning all the time about the effects and importance of minerals. Few minerals have figures for daily requirements which scientists, researchers and nutritionists will agree on. The major problem in working out such figures is that many quantities of the minerals eaten are simply not absorbed and used by the body. In a very complex action, many potentially rich minerals are never used to the full and are wasted. The minerals may be present in the food we eat, but fail to be absorbed into the blood stream.

And as if there were not enough threats to the poor minerals in their bid to bolster up our bodies, there is one more for us to look at – namely the way in which natural foods are altered. Over-cooking, preserving, freezing, canning, the addition of additives and colourings will all affect the quality of the food – and the benefit it has for us.

We all need certain amounts of each mineral; the problem is that these amounts differ. There is no set amount you should take – only limits. And the limits are there because too much can be as dangerous and as harmful as too little.

Selenium and the Perfect Diet

It is argued that a perfect diet will supply a man or woman with all the minerals that he or she needs. But how many are confident that their diet is perfect? Some people who have the time and the knowledge to reach that perfection of diet could sit back in complacency. Such people are few and far between and the vast majority of people in this country do not have a perfect diet. While the nation's eating habits may indeed be improving, there is still a long way to go; and even for those who are confident that their diet is such that nothing is lacking, here is something they might like to consider.

There is one mineral which your diet in the U.K. will not be able to provide enough of. There just is not enough of it in our soil. It was identified as a component of an organic constituent in 1957. Since then, eight other minerals have been linked to nutritional importance, although not one of them has caused similar world-wide scientific interest and genuine excitement. It has become something of a star personality in the mineral range and is named after the goddess of the moon – Selene. We know it as selenium.

2.

ASTOUNDING FACTS AND FIGURES

Selenium is no ordinary trace metal. Just for the record, let us get a few facts straight; selenium is a silver-grey element, has an atomic weight of 78.96, an atomic number of 34, a relative density of 4.81, and a melting point of 217°C. It also has the special property of conducting electricity when exposed to light and is therefore used in photo-electric cells. It is essential to the design of *Xerox* machines.

Selenium has the unusual feature of being distributed very unevenly in the earth's crust. This uneven distribution has meant that some communities have high and some low levels of the mineral. Almost all of Britain is in a low selenium belt. It has been this variation in the amount of selenium contained in different soils throughout the world which has helped studies trying to establish what the effects and the functions of the mineral are.

More research has gone into the nutritional value of selenium over the past twenty years than almost any other vitamin or mineral. In 1957, German-born physician, Klaus Schwartz, identified selenium as a compound of an

organic constituent he called Factor 3 which was very
successful in treating a dietary deficiency disease in rats.
Dr Schwartz had been working with several other potentially
important trace elements, including tin, vanadium and
nickel. But it was selenium which was to be the new hope
which attracted attention, and the basis of all that was
ahead in years of patient and painstaking work was the
recognition of the diet's important role in preventing
disease.

Developments in Veterinary Science
For a long time, the only evidence about selenium was
that in areas where levels in the soil were high, it
produced an intoxication in animals. It was then noted
that lower levels of selenium could prevent some of the
symptoms of vitamin E deficiency in animals. And it is
perhaps important to note that it was veterinary science
which first took a good hard look at selenium – for the
very commercial reason of improving livestock for the
market.

For many years, trace elements such as selenium were
given to domestic animals with dramatic results. In the
early 1970's, selenium was used in animal experiments
specializing in the study of ageing – under the heading of
anti-oxidants. It was found that the lifespan of rats and
mice was prolonged. A mouse normally lives for two
years, but with selenium added to the diet the lifespan is
increased to three years.

In 1973, the World Health Organization acknowledged
the growing amount of research throughout the world by
undertaking to study the effects of selenium in relation to
coronary heart disease. More and more studies in the
United States, Britain, Germany, Finland, New Zealand,
Russia, China, Japan, Canada, and elsewhere have meant
a growing wealth of information. The case now in favour
of selenium is overwhelming. For many years it has been
known to be essential to animals; now we know that the
human body needs it to be able to fight and conquer
illness.

Low Selenium Deposits

In 1977, something happened which startled many people
– and almost overnight convinced them of the importance
of selenium. It came in the form of a Government-
published report, under the direction of the Ministry of
Agriculture, Fisheries and Foods and what it said was that
there were not sufficient deposits of selenium in Britain's
soil to provide what we needed.

Selenium exists in small amounts in foods including
meat, seafood, wholegrain wheat, brewer's yeast, sesame
seeds, garlic, and mushrooms. The body only needs very
small amounts of selenium which is measured in millionths
of grams. But what was established was that those who
had been saying that a perfect diet would provide enough
selenium had been wrong. There just was not enough in
the soil for that to happen.

It was a problem which was getting worse, not better.
Artificial fertilizers were reducing the existing selenium
content and what was being taken out in this case could
not be put back. The dilemma was clear. Nutritionists
were saying on one hand that we needed certain levels of
this trace element. Yet if there was not enough selenium
in the soil, then there could not be enough in the crops or
livestock.

The irony was that the work into selenium by eminent
researchers was providing some of the most exciting facts
and findings possible. These facts linked low selenium
levels with high rates of heart disease and cancer, particularly breast cancer; it was found that selenium had a vital
role to play in the protection of each of the millions of
cells in the body, and could slow down the whole of the
body's ageing process.

In addition, it was shown that people were just not
getting enough selenium in their diet and that selenium
was able to combine with vitamin E in a vital way to
provide a powerful healing partnership for the body.
Research concluded that selenium could reduce the
threat of heavy metal poisoning and that modern processing
of foods was destroying this selenium content. It is these

facts and others which form the remarkable story which this book has to tell.

3.

A VICTORY
AGAINST ARTHRITIS

There is a natural cure for arthritis – and members of the
British Arthritic Association can prove it. They can prove
it because they are walking properly when once they used
to limp painfully and are now active and energetic when
once they were in considerable pain.

The role of selenium in providing relief from arthritis
has been known for some time. For many years animals
suffering from arthritis were given selenium combined
with vitamin E. The successes in those trials were considerable but the expected progression to see if the same
formula worked on human beings suffering from arthritis
was slow in coming.

But in 1982 there were two significant movements.

The first and the most dramatic featured a trial using
selenium on members of the British Arthritic Association.
The second was carried out by readers of *Here's Health*
magazine.

The results from both provided an insight into the way
the trace mineral can and does provide relief from a
disease which in its various forms is probably the most

widespread, crippling, disabling and painful in Britain.

The Arthritic Association selected some of their most chronic sufferers to take part in the trial. And they were prepared to do it because of the personal success story of Charles Ware, president of the Association who had almost 50 years of suffering from arthritis relieved by selenium.

'One of the effects', he said, 'was it removed a rash on my arms which has not come back except when I stopped taking selenium. But the main effect is on my hip. I have suffered for nearly 50 years from an arthritic hip and I have been trying to get rid of it for all these years but nothing cured it entirely.

'As a result of using selenium I have no pain whatsoever in my hip either at night or daytime and I have full movement of the leg.'

It was after this that he urged the Association to carry out a detailed trial.

He said it was important for the Association to put forward 'very bad cases'.

So the Arthritic Association decided at its council meeting on 22 April 1982 to carry out trials using Selenium on 100 patients who were 'suffering seriously with various forms of arthritis'. People on the trial started off with two tablets a day and then dropped to one tablet a day after a month.

The results were dramatically successful. Seven out of ten people said their arthritis and rheumatism had shown 'considerable improvement' from taking the selenium. Many admitted that painful hips and joints which had not responded to any other forms of treatments had been completely cured.

The results of the trial were presented in detail to the autumn meeting of the Arthritic Association. Almost immediately the product used in the trial – Selenium ACE – was added to the official list of remedial therapies for arthritis sufferers.

A spokesman for the association said after the trial: 'We as an association have always been keen to look at ways and treatments which will aid the relief available to those people suffering from arthritis. Our members who took part in the selenium trial have been thrilled by its success. There is no doubt it has brought help and in many cases has cured some of the most severe patients.

'We do believe that selenium has the potential to help many thousands of people who are victims of both rheumatism and arthritis. It is now one of our recommended treatments.' There is little doubt the trial by the British Arthritic Association represented a considerable breakthrough. Arthritis and rheumatism are so common that statistically, half the households in Britain have at least one sufferer. So, as an organization, the Arthritic Association is looking after the interests of a lot of people.

The success of selenium gave the Association the extra thrill of being a natural, drug-free product. A spokesman added: 'A lot of arthritis sufferers are concerned now about many of the drugs on the market. Recent publicity has left them reluctant to take risks with powerful drugs which have no proven success and often side-effects. There seems to be a much faster reaction from members about the success of a product against arthritis if it has the added benefit of being drug-free'.

The value of selenium against arthritis isn't new. It had its most dramatic successes in trials with animals. Tests on a wide variety of animals concentrated on using selenium with vitamin E. Yet strangely, despite an overwhelming success rate in relieving arthritic symptoms in sheep, dogs and other large animals, there was a reluctance to take the next step and see if the treatment worked with humans.

That reluctance is now over.

There are now three major trials planned for selenium and its anti-inflammatory properties to combat arthritis. One is in Japan, the second in California and the third planned for the Rheumatism and Arthritis Department of one of London's leading hospitals.

A lot of progress is being made generally in the understanding we have of arthritis. Increasing evidence

suggests that stress or poor diet can hinder recovery or
accentuate the problem. But regardless of the cause of
arthritis there is more evidence becoming available that
selenium, together with vitamin E, can give protection to
cells consistent with an anti-inflammatory effect. And it is
that protection that could account for reduced pain and
disappearance of symptoms.

Veterinarians have found that arthritic pain and swellings
can be controlled with a mixture of selenium and vitamin
E. What has been used in the treatment of animals is a
product which contains between 60 and 70 international
units of vitamin E and 1000 micrograms of selenium. At
the Animal Research Laboratory at Boston City Hospital
in the United States in 1982 trials were carried out on a
group of dogs with severe joint swellings. The pre-trial
condition of the animals was said to be 'serious' with
many of them crippled. The results of the four-month
trial using selenium with vitamin E were again enormously
successful with 70 per cent of the dogs responding to
treatment. One third of the animals taking the mixture
over a longer period had the symptoms 'improved considerably'.

The trial highlighted something else. Many of the
animals were found to have low blood selenium levels.
This discovery supported research work in May 1980 in
Norway where a rheumatoid arthritis group had shown
very low levels of selenium in their blood. They too were
treated with selenium and vitamin E. The results showed
that pain in a large number of the group was reduced.

At any given time throughout the world literally
hundreds of hospitals, clinics and research centres are
concentrating on finding the successful path to bring
relief to rheumatism and arthritis. Selenium is only one of
many such paths. But there have been so many positive
results using the trace mineral that it is now being
acknowledged as one of the most exciting developments
in recent years.

So how is it that the combined effect of selenium with
vitamin E has caused so much genuine excitement in the

world of medical research?

Let's first look at both arthritis and rheumatism and how they can cripple and injure.

Arthritis is a word that comes from the Greek, *arthron* – joint and *itis* – inflammation. It is quite literally an inflamed joint. Although arthritis is almost accepted now as a description of any ache or pain it should properly be reserved for cases involving joints. Rheumatism is now more identified with a condition which includes painful joints, ligaments, tendons and muscles.

Osteo-arthritis is the most wide-spread form of the arthritic diseases. It is a slow disorder characterized by a breakdown of cartilage and changes in the bone. It develops more often than not in the fingers and in the joints of the body which have to carry weight – the knees, the hips and the spine. The joint effect of these collective group of diseases has been nothing short of appalling in terms of pain and illnesses all over the world. Certainly arthritis shows no mercy in terms of individual pain to millions – or in the cost to the country in lost working hours and in National Health Service expenditure.

The exact cause of rheumatoid arthritis is not known. There may not be any single cause. One of the longest established views is that arthritis is the result of some sort of infection. As yet no infectious agent has been singled out. Researchers increasingly believe that the painful changes in the joints may be due to some toxic infection elsewhere in the body. It may be a question of mineral deficiencies in the blood stream and shortages of certain important vitamins have also been suspected.

The question of stress cannot be ignored and, while clearly not the principal cause, is seen as weakening the resistance of the body as does a lot of physical strain and regularly letting joints become exposed to cold and damp. In most cases the arthritis will appear gradually. It may be a question of soreness and stiffness of swelling in a joint for several weeks. Then other joints become involved and there are increasingly a number of changes in the body. The fingers and toes are commonly involved.

Oddly, rheumatoid arthritis often singles out the middle joints while osteo-arthritis normally develops first in the end joints. It has been important to look at the disease and to see how widespread it is to put into context some of the excitement now being generated by selenium and the way the trace element works synergistically with such vitamins as vitamins C, E and A.

There has, for some years now, been some significance in the relationship of various trace minerals in the body and the person who is suffering from arthritis. The role of selenium, manganese and zinc have been isolated from the complicated chain reactions of the blood cells from people known to be suffering from arthritis.

It was only the revealing series of tests which showed such a low level of selenium present in the blood of a large number of arthritic patients in both Norway and the United States that the right sort of questions began to be asked.

And if, as some researchers believe, arthritis is caused by an as yet unknown virus, the body's defence against such a virus would consist of protective blood cells as well as antibodies. It is the role of trace elements in those blood cells and in the complicated reaction of dangerous enzymes that much investigation is centering on. We have highlighted elsewhere in this book the fact that selenium itself is of little value by itself. You have to have one or two vitamins to activate it and bring it to life. Certainly the role of vitamin E is critical.

There are literally thousands of reports in medical literature which show that heart conditions and many other circulatory problems improve with doses of vitamin E. Now researchers in the United States and in Japan believe the vitamin to be effective in preventing the bone softening and the frequent bone fractures that often go side by side with the administration of many steroid drugs. Its role with selenium is now being tested again in Moscow. Fresh work will be concentrated on the way they link together in one specific enzyme in the body. What is clear is that the trace mineral combined with the remarkable properties of vitamin E are a powerful 'team' together. The way they link could go part of the way to an explanation of the relief being brought to arthritic sufferers.

One final and important vitamin needs to be considered in the jigsaw puzzle. And that is vitamin C. Research into vitamin C and the prevention of colds is now well established. Less accepted is its role as an anti-inflammatory agent. As long ago as 1971 researchers noted in *The Lancet* medical journal a study of how aspirin destroys vitamin C in the body. Arthritics are generally deficient in this particular vitamin. Aspirin for many sufferers is the principal weapon in their fight against arthritis. A significant link was formed. Inflammatory disorders have now been identified as reacting positively to large doses of vitamin C – disorders like bursitis, tendonitis and, yes, arthritis.

It is known that vitamin C performs many functions inside the body and that it takes part in many enzyme systems which control the way we use this or that nutrient. Increasingly vitamin C has been one of the vitamins thought to be another of the triggering mechanisms for selenium, with vitamin E seen as an important addition.

The story isn't over yet. In fact it may be that it has only just begun. The whole success that selenium is now having with arthritic patients is gaining worldwide attention. Major symposiums reviewing and updating research on selenium will now be annual events. One leading American researcher, Dr E. J. Crary, said recently that the nutritional importance of selenium was increasing year by year:

'Of course we have to temper our enthusiasm by seeking the proper sorts of clinical trials. There is so much evidence now that we need, almost internationally, to decide on an ordered programme of research which will cover the way selenium reacts within our bodies.' He also highlighted the way it has worked with arthritis patients.

In the autumn of 1982 one of Canada's leading arthritis

research clinics decided to study many of the trace minerals and their reaction as anti-inflammatory agents. Gold, zinc and selenium were singled out and a paper prepared which came out in favour of a major controlled trial on selenium.

'What we have been able to do', said the report, 'is to identify the major potential selenium may have in combatting many of the symptoms we now commonly link together as being arthritic. The sort of investigations we now call for have been beyond the scope of our research but we believe them to be of importance.'

Such research may now be pioneered in Japan. Kyoto's University Medical Research Unit which has some of the most modern research facilities in the world has been conducting research into the effects of minerals from the soil. They have concentrated on the way food grown in different soils can have different properties. What the initial findings have shown is that selenium levels can be critical to health both in general and in specific terms. A programme is now being started to look at selenium's role as a natural cure for arthritis.

So the next two or three years may yet reveal some of the answers. What has been established is that selenium can bring relief to arthritis. It can do it not in the way of a drug. There is no overnight cure. Indeed many of the people who have had joints cured from arthritic pain have noted a slight initial increase in swelling or an increase in pain. This is by no means true in every case but looking through the comments made by people on the trial by the arthritic association it is something that crops up. There seems to be a reaction and then without fail the symptoms start to ease.

How long is it before there is a lessening in the pain? Again there is no exact time which can be laid down. It isn't an instant success – but it is a course of treatment which needs to be continued for a minimum of four to six weeks. Some of the people taking part in the Arthritic Association trial were, as we have seen, severe cases. The selenium trial was for 90 days. Many extended it. At the

90 day period the pain was lessened but not gone completely. The extended course improved many conditions even more.

Selenium isn't a pain killer. There won't be instant relief. The inter-reaction of the selenium with the other vitamins does take time. The signs are that it can stop the acceleration of the disease – and then work on healing. And it won't work for everyone. But when 1,000 readers of *Here's Health* magazine tested the product in 1982 it worked for almost nine out of ten of them in some way. A large proportion of them noted the benefit it had for arthritic complaints. Others said that it had helped their general health, headaches, hypertension and circulation complaints. Some of their comments are included at the end of this book.

Here's Health readers gave their verdict in much the same way as the people involved in the arthritic association had done. Neither test was clinically controlled in any way. Such controlled trials will now form part of future research. What the two tests in 1982 did was to give some indication that people could find help in selenium for arthritis. It was also seen by those who remain convinced of the properties of the mineral that it can no longer be ignored in serious research terms. I have spoken to some of the people who have had crippling arthritis who have known the despair it can bring. They were some of the worst cases which the British Arthritic Association put forward for the selenium trial. Of those people two stories stand out.

The first concerns a 61-year-old woman called Joyce. She had been a member of the Arthritic Association for five years and was keen to take up the offer to try selenium. Her reason was simple. She would try anything that gave her some hope. Arthritis had started in her left hip and had become so bad that she was restricted to her chair. She slept in the downstairs lounge because she couldn't get up her stairs. Doctors and specialists had gone through the progression of drugs – including Opren – and had warned about a hip replacement operation.

Selenium hadn't had any effect to start with. It was six weeks into the treatment when she noticed something. 'The hip was still painful but I had been getting pain in my fingers and that started to get a lot better. Then over the next few weeks it became less and less painful. I began to walk a bit. I managed to walk upstairs and round the corner.' The pain hasn't completely disappeared. She admits to twinges. 'It isn't the severe pain I had before. There's still a lot of discomfort but selenium has been wonderful. I don't know whether I could have lived with the pain for much longer. It has meant so much to me.'

The second case worth mentioning is a man whose hands were crippled with arthritis. Again drugs had shown no help and other joints were painful. He spoke of the depression which had come about because he could see that nothing would help him.

'I was resigned to it. My hands were the worst. I just couldn't control them. When I tried selenium I had some swelling and I almost gave up after three or four weeks. I've tried so many things that people have told me would work only to be disappointed, that I thought this would be another one. Then the feelings came back into my hands and fingers and it's really been wonderful. It has, I believe, cured me.'

4.

THE SUCCESS STORIES

For all the explanation and evidence that is constantly being sifted out there remains one fact that no-one can deny. And that is simply that a large number of people who have taken selenium to fight arthritis have found success and relief from pain.

The words of this particular chapter are the words of the people who have found that relief. These are only a small number of the many who have offered their thoughts after taking selenium on trial. Specifically they come from those who took part in the British Arthritic Association trial and in the tests carried out by *Here's Health* magazine readers.

*   *   *

'I don't trust drugs so I won't take them. I have had very painful knees for many years and they often get stiff. I've been taking selenium for the 90 day period and my knees feel a lot better now. They still seem to click now and again when I move quickly but there's not a fraction of the pain there used to be.'

* * *

'I have suffered with rheumatic pain in my neck and left shoulder for about three years but since taking the selenium I've had no pain now for two months. Thank you so much.'

* * *

'I had been taking Methrazone and Opren at one time for my arthritis. At first I felt worse taking selenium. I had been taking the drugs for two and a half years. The selenium seemed to give me aches all over. Then the pain started to disappear and after two months I began to feel very much better than I have done for the past seven years.'

* * *

'My joint pains eased after approximately four weeks but the muscular pain and stiffness took six to eight weeks before improvement. My enlarged joints have now reduced to almost normal and I shall go on taking selenium.'

* * *

'I had a very painful lump at the side of my knee. After a month of taking the selenium it went. I tried drugs but they didn't have any effect. I was told to take selenium and be patient. It wouldn't clear it overnight someone told me, but it would cure it. I've recommended it for a lot of people I know who suffer from arthritis.'

* * *

'I sent for these tablets (selenium) thinking I had arthritis in my hand which I had smashed at the beginning of the year. It turned out to be rheumatic fever. I honestly don't think I would be here now if it hadn't been for these pills. My heart is still bad and my blood-pressure higher than I thought but I'm mending well and I shall go on taking selenium.'

*   *   *

'I have had hip arthritis which just got worse and worse as my weight increased. The pain was just terrible. I was so scared about the publicity given to some of the drugs that all I used to take was an aspirin now and again when it became too much to bear. I tried taking selenium and it seemed that for the first week my joints flared up. Then there wasn't as much pain. It was one weekend after I had been taking the tablets for about eight weeks when I realized the pain was completely gone. It was wonderful – thank you.'

*   *   *

'After a coronary four years ago I know I have a slightly raised blood-pressure and possible hardening of the arteries. I have also had a lot of pain in an arthritic knee. I had to use a walking stick and to an extent I was becoming a cripple with it. The pain some days was more than I could bear. The articles I have read on selenium have made a big impression. I tried the tablets and I have no pain in my knee. It stiffens up sometimes but that soon disappears. I shall continue to take them in the belief that they will help me for the rest of my life.'

*   *   *

'For the first four weeks no improvement. After that each day the pain in my hand, arm and shoulder started to ease up. My headaches vanished. Then I could get my arm higher and higher. Now I can do my polishing with my right arm, stretch to do my windows. I now only get a small twinge occasionally if I polish too heavily. My arm is quite mobile again (no crying with the dreadful pain). Also my nails have stopped breaking and they are quite strong. I have even enrolled for a keep fit class.'

*   *   *

'I have had arthritis for six years. I take a pain killer for my shoulder which is the worst place. I couldn't lift it at all. My legs were starting to get worse. I only live fifty yards from the shops but I couldn't walk there any more. My neighbour had to do all the shopping. I tried the selenium tablets and I was disappointed when nothing happened for week after week. Then after about two months the pain started to ease. I've been taking them for almost four months now. My legs are much better and I can walk really well and lift my shoulder. It has made life worthwhile again.'

5.

CAN YOU REALLY STAY YOUNGER LONGER?

The name Leon Ojeda probably will not mean very much to you; neither will Miguel Carpio. They are by no means famous names or faces, but both have lived in remote areas of South America for a very very long time. Evidence which has been checked and cross-checked suggests that Leon was over 130 years old. Miguel claimed to be 123, but a series of cross-checks revealed that somewhere he had lost track of the years. He was in fact 129. Both men lived in the Andean highlands where communities have been reaching ages which consistently top the 100 year mark. These people grow old, yet still remain agile and lucid. Death from cancer or heart disease is unknown to such communities.

The two men lived in the Vilcabamba Valley in Ecuador – one of three increasingly famous areas of the world where great age has become a subject of intense study. The other two areas are the Southern Caucasus of the Soviet Union and the Hunza section of Pakistan which links China, Pakistan and the Soviet Union. In these three areas, people live longer than anywhere else in the world.

Longevity in Ecuador

A growing number of scientists and researchers have
spent many months with the people from these areas.
One such man was Dr David Davies from the Gerontological Unit of University College, London. He found
that the centenarians in Ecuador provided the blueprint
for a study in depth. The hundreds of certificates he saw
he accepted as being undoubtedly genuine. He found
death certificates of four people who lived to 150 years
and died in the 1920's and 1930's. There were baptismal
certificates for people in the region of 120 and 130 years
of age. What the certificates showed him – and they were
verified and checked by village priests – was that there was
a pattern, a pattern of great age.

This remarkable occurrence of longevity was linked
with a total absence of the killer diseases of cancer and of
the heart. Yet among infants, about 40 per cent died
before they reached their fourth year; succumbing to the
usual epidemics and viruses. In the growing up process,
they became immune to many of the diseases and after
their teens seemed very physically hardy.

The diet of these South Americans living in the valleys
was austere and monotonous. They were, and still are,
very poor people and live on green vegetables, cabbages,
marrows, pumpkins and fruit. In addition, maize, soya
beans, cottage cheese made from cows' or goats' milk and
eggs – either eaten raw or almost raw – supplement the
diet. Almost no one eats meat.

The growing and picking of herbs are part of the way of
life, and the people have a deep knowledge and understanding of the plants and herbal remedies which are used
for everything from increasing the fertility of cattle to
healing skin complaints; from smallpox outbreaks to
curing baldness. It is a way of life, of eating, which
nutritionists believe holds the key to the great and almost
unbelievable ages that are being reached.

Yet you only have to move away from these wild and
primitive areas, away from the valley to nearby towns and
villages, to find things change dramatically. For in those

towns the diet is based on much more refined foods –
pasta, white flour, white sugar and tinned foods. It is far
removed from the austere mountain and valley diet, and
the fact that the health of the centenarians is not threatened
by cancer, heart disease and diabetes is all the more
remarkable since, in the nearby towns and villages, these
diseases are common.

Centenarians in Russia
But the phenomenon of longevity is not confined to this
one South American valley. The Russians, only quite
recently, began to show interest in the fact that some of
their people were living to great ages. At present, a special
Institute of Gerontology is working on research into men
such as Shirali Luslimov who, until his death in 1973, was
the oldest person in this southern region of Russia. One
of his brothers died at the age of 134 and another brother
of 106 also lived in the same village. The village is in the
mountains of Azerbaijan, near the Russo-Iranian border,
a very similar setting and way of life to that which Dr
Davies found in Ecuador.

Research in the region by eminent Russion, French
and American scientists has produced some facts. A study
on one village in the region, with a population of 1,200,
showed there were 71 men and 110 women between the
ages of 81 and 90. Nineteen were over 90. Only the
slightest signs of heart disease were found and there were
no reported cases of cancer in a nine-year study of 123
people, said to be over 100 years of age. The Abkhasian
people, originally nomads, eat hardly any meat. Fresh
fruit and vegetables such as beans, onions and many root
vegetables play an important part in their diet. They are
great eaters of garlic and sugar is never eaten.

The Hunzas of Pakistan
The last of this trio of areas which has caused such
amazing instances of old age is in northern Pakistan
where the Hunza people live. Again, it is a similar setting –
remote and difficult to reach. The area has become

politically difficult for scientists and researchers to reach.
It sits in a sensitive corner of the world, nestled between
Pakistan, the Soviet Union and China. But even so, the
research that has been possible shows that many men
have lived to be 120.

To the Hunzas, care of the land is the most important
thing in their lives. They live on food, mostly grain, green
vegetables and root vegetables, grown in their own soil.
Pulses form a vital part of their diet. The lack of meat-
eating is caused by the fact that they are so poor. These
people also exercise a great deal, never retire and have no
such childhood diseases as mumps, chicken-pox or
measles. In the adult population there are no known
cancer cases.

Old age is thought by some to run in families, and it is
clearly true that this may be a factor. But there is an
important difference to note between some of the centenarians of the three areas of the world we have been
looking at. If living to great age means the loss of most of
the faculties – as it often does in the U.K. – then the
prospect of getting very old has very little glamour or
appeal attached to it. The great ages we have highlighted
feature people who have never retired and who have
stayed healthy and active. They go on playing an important
role in the community in which they live. In such regions,
there is no question of early retirement and perhaps
ending their days in an old people's home; this represents
a great difference in lifestyles.

The Ageing Process
In all the recent research into what happens when people
grow old, there have been very few discoveries which
indicate that something has gone wrong with the body
simply because of the passage of time. What we can say is
that ageing is the process which reduces the number of
healthy cells in the body. What happens is that although
the systems in the body continue to perform, the first
thing to suffer is the back-up systems which are often
called upon to come to the rescue. The body's loss of

reserve is due to the decreasing amount of cells in each organ. The reduction in the number of cells in our bodies actually begins before we are born and it sets the pattern for our lifestyle – and the ageing process that we have to come to terms with. The way our cells – and there are 60,000 billion of them – cope with day to day life is affected by chemical reactions, not by the passage of the years. Therefore, if it is possible to have some control over those reactions, is it then possible to slow down the whole process which governs the rate at which we grow older?

Scientists studying the ageing process for the past twenty years have found that there are two basic processes. One is the basic ageing pattern and the loss of healthy cells itself. The second is dictated by the way we live, where we live and how much we allow our bodies to be abused. Status and lifestyle, the importance of diet and exercise and other things can cause the whole ageing process to accelerate ten to twenty years earlier than it would under different circumstances. Your body will literally grow older faster because of the way you live. Add to these factors the very real dangers of early retirement where the mind and body change down several gears and a 'lazier' lifestyle may be adopted, then the process is accelerated again.

If the way we live controls the ageing process, then what is it about the way we live which is so important? In South America, in regions of the Soviet Union and Pakistan the common factor is the diet. It is a diet low in calories and protein and is very closely linked to the soil, in which all the food is grown. These may turn out to be the crucial factors. The connection with the soil is important because it relates to discoveries made about trace elements, particularly in Ecuador – trace minerals known to be needed by the body.

Lifestyle also plays a crucial role. The long-lived people of the remote regions all stay busy on the land. The body is made to work, and work hard, at ages where, in other countries, it is a time when there is little to do but sit and sleep. No one is suggesting that these centenarians are freaks. They can no longer live life at a great pace, but the difference is that they have succeeded in slowing down the whole process of ageing more than any other people on earth.

Diet and Old Age

Research in less obscure areas, noteably in the West, has noted the longevity of vegetarians whose diets, usually of necessity, fall somewhat short in protein. Thomas Parr, the Englishman who lived for 152 years, was a vegetarian. So were George Bernard Shaw, Bernard MacFadden and many other noteable people who lived to be very old. They also remained free of cancer and serious illnesses. A study of the diet of American black people revealed that, on average, they ate much less protein than American whites. Their diet was much more basic, with fewer processed and more home-grown foods. The study showed that blacks are living longer and that they suffer far less from major stomach diseases.

The food we eat, its calorie and protein content and where it comes from are now accepted as forming part of the second process which controls the way we age. Laboratory tests have cut the amounts of proteins and calories given to rats and mice – and, in such cases, they have lived longer. It is now being predicted that the right sort of diet could increase the period of adult vigour by 20 per cent, as long as it is started early enough.

Perhaps the most illuminating study done in the United States was the one carried out by Dr Roland Phillips, who compared the diets and cancer rates of two religious groups – Seventh Day Adventists and Mormons. Both of these groups have turned their backs totally on smoking and alcohol and both promote and pursue a very similar lifestyle. There are two significant differences. Seventh Day Adventists do not generally eat meat; Mormons do. In addition, there is a group of Mormons who live in a rather special area of Utah, the significance of which will soon be seen. At a special symposium on nutrition and cancer Dr Phillips presented his research which showed that the non-meat eating Seventh Day Adventists experience a much lower cancer rate than the meat-eating Mormons. What is also showed was that the Mormons who lived in and around Utah were much less likely to be affected by cancer than other members of their group living elsewhere. And the significance of Utah is that it is one of the States to have a high deposit of selenium in the soil, something which was isolated as being of importance in the statistics.

The Role of Trace Elements

In the research into longevity, one of the most exciting single factors has now been agreed. It is the existence of trace elements found in the soil, water and diet. Samples of water and soil taken from the Vilcabamba mountains and valleys showed that the water was very pure with hardly any minerals in it. The soil, on the other hand, was full of minerals. The great areas for long life in the world are all areas surrounded by high mountains, so that the trace elements are leached off the higher ground and deposited in large quantities in the valleys. It is those minerals which find their way into the body by passing from the soil into the food we eat. The evidence is still being gathered, but Dr Davies has said: 'The effects of trace elements on bodily health and function are significant, as may be the interplay of various trace elements upon each other. Certainly it is true that there was a marked pinkish colouration of the soil where we found these pockets of longevity. And the striking and extreme tooth decay found among these people may well be connected with the action of rare trace elements – and the fact that longevity and this unusual tooth decay exist side by side is fascinating. It may lead us to some important conclusions. Since working in this area I have discussed the problem of trace elements with several scientists and believe that it is possible that there is some rare trace element reaction. These trace elements are an exciting discovery.'

Norfolk's Selenium Deposits

A 1977 report from the Ministry of Agriculture, Fisheries and Food revealed that large areas of England are low in selenium. There is only one selenium-rich region where glacial action millions of years ago left deposits of this important mineral in adequate quantities. And in that one area of North Norfolk, near the popular holiday town of Sheringham, there are two to three times as many people over 75 years of age as in the country as a whole. In Norwich, 11 per cent of the people are 75 years old or older, and in Upper Sheringham and nearby, 15 per cent are over 75. The national average shows that only five per cent of the population lives over the magic 75 years of age.

There are certain similarities between the people who live in this unique corner of Britain and the other more dramatic areas for longevity. The principal one is that much of the food eaten is grown locally and fresh fruit and vegetables form the basis of the diet. There is also the other link with the land – the area still remains pre-dominantly agricultural. But if you are thinking of selling up and moving to a longer, richer life by living in this part of Norfolk, then there is a word of warning – it is not that simple. Certainly it is an ideal situation to live in a selenium-rich area, but you have got to build up your bodily intake. Estimates are that you need to live in such an area for at least eight years before the increased selenium intake begins to produce any noticeable improvement to health.

However, for the people living there, selenium has caused some rather unusual problems. Bill Sutton, for example, has for the most part been quite happy as secretary to his local over 70's club. He helped to start the club, but now it has become more trouble to him than it is worth. The problem is that there are too many people who want to join and consequently there is now a ban on new members.

Bill, who is well into his late 70's said: 'We had over 90 active members who all seemed to want to come to all our meetings and trips. More and more heard about us and wanted to come along. But we have not got the room so we said no to any more joining and since then a lot of them have been getting quite nasty about it. I just say it is not my fault.'

The problem is that it is not just a case of the people living in this area living longer; they tend to be more active as well. One of the characters of the area is 96 year-old Billy Collins who cycles every day round the village of Bodham and West Backham. His wife Amy still runs a thriving vegetable produce stall outside their cottage. Amy does all the gardening and she is 91 years old. Her next-door neighbour and best friend is 85. When Billy goes down to the pub, two of his drinking mates are 87 and 84. The area has been known in the past few years to boast three active centenarians. Mary Dunne who is 82 and runs the entertainments section for the Darby and Joan club, where the average age is 74, said:

'I don't think we think of it as being a special place. There are a lot of elderly people but they all seem sprightly and well. I think it's a very happy and active place to live. We're close to the sea and there's some lovely walks, so I suppose people think that helps to keep us all healthy. It's true that most people grow their own vegetables. I think you have to. It's a way of getting cheap food.'

Lifespan and Selenium

Increasingly, research work is now aimed at studying the effect on lifespan of selenium soil levels. It is now believed that selenium is one of the most vital elements to come from the soil and one of the key roles it plays is in reducing the damage that accelerates the ageing process. In the same way, selenium deficiency can age you faster. The recommended amount will ensure that your body can develop the ability to keep the ageing rate down. One estimate has put the difference down to as much as ten to 15 years of healthy life. So if the average lifespan is, say, 70 then it could and should be increased to as much as 85.

So where's the proof? In the late 1960's, experiments began on selenium because it was thought that as a compound it might be able to work synergistically with other compounds known to extend the lifespan. It had earlier been established that vitamin E and a few synthetic antioxidants extended the average lifespan of mice and rats.

Trials on small animals have taken a wide variety of diets and applied them over a long period. Rats fed for 27 months (the rough equivalent of 50 years in human terms) on a diet similar to that of the Hunza region and consisting of chapattis made of wholemeal flour, pulses, raw carrots, unboiled milk and water showed that none of the animals became ill, and all survived to a ripe old age. Richer foods, processed with more calories, shortened life and led to greater outbreaks of disease.

It was established that the fewer calories rats were given, the longer they lived. So the theory began to evolve that a correct diet could prolong life – a theory which has now become more prominent and better established in recent years than ever before.

Experiments by Dr Richard Passwater went a stage further than the initial work done on vitamin E. It had been shown that selenium did work with some of the functions of vitamin E and the relationship between the 'vitality vitamin' and selenium was to take on greater significance in other work. Dr Passwater included selenium in a series of tests with antioxidants. In a long catalogue of experiments with mice he was able to successfully develop a range of antioxidant compounds which added 20 to 30 per cent to the mean lifespan. Two years after that, the combinations in which selenium played such a vital role produced lifespan increases of 175 per cent. They were a crucial series of tests in the development of the under-standing of selenium and its role in the ageing process.

Defence Against Cell Damage
Another major theory which contributed to the under-standing of selenium and the ageing process also came

from Dr Passwater and concerned the role of free radicals in the body. Free radicals are highly reactive fragments of molecules in the body, which can cause damage by destroying cells. Because they are highly reactive, they can start off a link system and form stronger and stronger chains, eventually being released to destroy body components. So these incomplete molecules can do considerable damage to the body cells. Five basic types of damage, including membrane damage, were isolated and free radicals were found to be the cause. What was damaged above all was the ability of the cell membrane to take in nutrients and to expel or get rid of toxic wastes. The whole cell chemistry was seen to be affected.

However, there is in the body a defence mechanism against these attacks. It comes in the form of enzymes or groups of proteins which act as catalysts. One of those enzymes is called glutathione peroxide, which contains atoms of selenium. So selenium was identified as a key compound in the body's in-built defence against cell damage, cell damage which accelerated the ageing process.

Yet despite studies in special gerontological centres in various areas, there has been criticism that not enough laboratory experiments have been done. Most scientists use small animals to test their theories. If positive results are found in mice, can the same results be applied in the case of man? The adaptation of such long-term tests on human beings in clinical trials presents unique problems. Nevertheless, there is growing agreement that ageing is a combination of cell loss and the production of improper enzymes and cells – both caused by free radical reactions. Selenium has a role to play in combating those reactions.

Dr Passwater's findings on selenium were put to the test in trials measuring the body's age pigment. Three diets were used in the trials on mice; one fortified with vitamin E, the second containing even more vitamin E and extra vitamin C, and the third included everything tested in the other two, plus selenium. The selenium diet drastically reduced the accumulation of the age pigment, seen to be as good as any of the ways of judging the process of life. The results implied that fewer cells had been destroyed and the ageing process had been slowed down in comparison to less protected animals.

No one is saying that selenium will make you younger; it is no witches' brew. What it does mean is that if you fail to get the amount of selenium that your body needs, then it will not have full protection against the complex ageing processes that have taken place within your system since before you were born. The danger is that you will become older than your years. Work on the effects selenium has on the whole ageing process is continuing and nutritionists are clearly excited by some of the developments.

One vital factor may be the link between growing older and the dangers of contracting disease. There is a strong link between most types of cancer and age. It is thought that cancer may appear in older people because it takes decades for some cancers to develop. More recent studies have indicated that the ageing process of the body makes people more vulnerable to cancer. So if the process can be slowed down, the body may become less vulnerable to cancer and other major diseases. Thus we shall live longer and better lives.

6.

FIGHTING CANCER NATURALLY

Let's start with the bad news: For men living in Britain today, the odds are that one in four will develop cancer. Of those, one in 30 will get cancer of the lung and one in 35 will get cancer of the stomach. If you are a woman, one in five will get cancer, of which one in 20 will have cancer of the breast. These are fairly depressing statistics. Certainly the word cancer probably provokes more anxiety and fear than any other ailment or disease in our society. It can strike at any age and is the second most common cause of death in the Western world. Only heart disease claims more lives.

In the past, cancer was invariably fatal. To be told you had cancer was a death sentence. Myths, half truths and misconceptions have built up almost inevitably as medical progress has been made towards the control and greater understanding of the disease. The truth is that progress is slow, giant strides towards conquering cancer are rare and many have been false alarms. Yet despite this, modern treatment which has become increasingly sophisticated and complex is helping thousands and thousands of people with different forms of cancer. Diet, nutrition, herbs, laetrile, megavitamin therapy have all made moves in the past towards offering a natural alternative to the control of cancer.

The weight of research behind these and many other theories makes it increasingly difficult to find the areas where real progress is being made. Now and again one theory is given a large amount of publicity, creates an interest and then fades into the background. Such 'break-throughs' are seldom borne out by the reality of the situation and so it all ends up in a confusing picture.

Orthodox methods of treating cancer still forge ahead in terms of development and research. And while, in the last ten years, the natural alternatives have captured more and more attention throughout the world, it is worth stressing that no one under-estimates the word cancer. And those who actively promote and encourage wider knowledge and research into the nutritional therapies are among the first to recommend a doctor's advice. No one is naive enough to suggest that a 'do-it-yourself' remedy is available without expert medical help and attention.

What is Cancer?

The word cancer was originally used to describe a range of infections and malignancies. It is derived from the French word *cancre* which became known in England as canker. Now we accept cancer in its basic sense as the uncontrollable growth of cells which develop from uncontrolled changes or mutations in the genetic material in a single cell. The important words are 'uncontrolled growth'. There are three basic types of cancer – carcinomas, sarcomas and leukaemia-like cancers. The changes in the genetic material result in cell growth that does not respond to normal controls within the body; and that is the difference between cancer, or a malignant growth, and a benign growth. For instance, when you cut yourself the skin cells receive impulses or signals to divide and repair the injury. When the injury has been repaired, signals are sent out to repair cell growth. But the cancer cell does not obey the normal laws. They not only grow and continue growing out of control, but also spread to other parts of the body and eventually work a complex passage into the organs.

The majority of cancers are caused, it is increasingly believed, by chemical damage to cell membranes which leads to cell mutation. A mutated cell in the body grows or divides and can lead to fully fledged cancer. The cell membrane is like an outer casing which protects the cell and, at the same time, carries nutrients into and waste products out of it. When the cell casing becomes damaged for any reason, then goodness cannot find its way in and the cell may well die.

Normal cells stop growing when they meet neighbouring cells but, unlike the case of the cut finger, the cancer cells refuse to react that way. They keep on growing uncontrollably. This type of cell membrane damage arises from the activity of the free radicals, fragments of molecules which can form their own chain reactions. It is the reaction of these free radicals to something known as DNA which is the critical factor. DNA is deoxyribonucleic acid and is the matter in living material that reproduces itself and forms all the materials and the cells of the human body. There is one important exception in DNA; the 45 essential nutrients can be taken into the body one and one way only – through the diet. Of those 45 or so essential nutrients, about 15 are minerals.

Reducing the Risk of Cancer

Free radicals are produced in the body as a matter of routine. They can be and are held in check by anti-radical elements or antioxidants such as vitamins A, C, E and minerals, notably selenium. Currently very exciting evidence suggests that improved selenium nutrition can reduce the risk of cancer. In recent studies, tests were carried out on animals treated with cancer-causing substances. Amounts of selenium were added to the diets and, in almost every case, selenium supplementation reduced the incidence of cancer. Scientists believe that the theory behind the potential success or scope for success of the trace element is very sound; and the more the theory has been explored, the more fascinating and exciting the potential seems to be. The clue that we all need a source of dietary selenium is to be found in the knowledge of the biochemical role of the element in tissues.

One of the best known studies has been carried out by Dr Gerhard N. Schrauzer, Prof. of Chemistry at the University of California. He has become well known for his championing of the cause of selenium. In one study he featured a controlled group of mice which had been seen to develop breast cancer spontaneously. The figures speak for themselves. Among the group which did not receive extra selenium, 83 per cent developed breast cancer. The mice whose diets were boosted by having extra selenium throughout their lives lived longer and developed cancer in only 10 per cent of the cases. Dr Schrauzer became involved in the study of breast cancer because, as he says, it is the most common cancer in women. He stressed it was an important cancer because it affected women in the prime of their lives and health. According to his studies, although breast cancer is now a universal disease, there are populations of women who show greater liability to develop it – and earlier in their lives.

In Japan, for instance, the incidence of breast cancer is far less than in the United States. However, if Japanese women emigrate to the United States their incidence of breast cancer rises; and it rises to such an alarming extent that, by the second generation, the Japanese-American woman has the same risk of developing the disease as the American woman. Schrauzer also high-lighted Yugoslavia as an area where breast cancer is very similar to that found in Japan. There are few easily identifiable links between the two countries.

He developed the thinking that there were 'laws' behind the different relative high and low incidences of cancer. The common link was diet. The next stage of the jigsaw puzzle was to look at the consumption of different foods. To start with, he looked at how much meat and how much bread was being eaten. And what was shown was that the higher the standard of living, the more meat featured in the diet – and the less important became foods such as bread and cereals. 'As we start to eat less cereals, so it seems that the cancer mortality goes up'. He expanded the research until it got to the stage where he was working on the theory that eating fat and meat increased the probability of cancer occurring, while eating bread, cereals and fish lowered the chances. So what was the precious ingredient which was able to offer some sort of protection against cancer?

Trace Elements and Cancer

To try and find the answer Dr Schrauzer switched his attention to a specific area of the human diet – trace elements and trace minerals. Of all the trace elements, selenium appeared to be the most prominent because of the wide variation in its intake. He was able to show that there was an inverse relationship between the availability of the selenium and how much cancer was identified. The more selenium there was in the diet, the less cancer there was.

As these studies were taking place, research in New Zealand where selenium intakes are low had shown that by giving an increased amount of the trace element to sheep, the incidence of sheep cancer was almost totally eradicated. But Dr Schrauzer has been carrying out tests since the mid-1960's. In 1971, he reported that one of the blood tests for cancer was actually a test for blood selenium level. He then linked the low levels of selenium with the greatest susceptibility to cancer. Dr Schrauzer and his colleagues developed the work to a major study to find where selenium levels were high and low – and how it translated into the occurrence of cancer. In 27 countries they found that the cancer death rate was inversely proportional to the dietary intake of selenium in the typical diets of those countries. Cancers involved in the studies included tumours of the breast, ovary, colon,

rectum as well as leukaemia. Another study showed that
the blood selenium levels of people from 17 of those
countries were also inversely proportional to the breast
cancer rate. The more selenium found naturally in the
soil, the lower was the chance of cancer.

One of the London hospitals which has spent much
time on research into selenium and in particular the
effect it can have on cancer produced a further encouraging
report in late 1982. The Laboratory of Pharmacokinetics
and Toxicology, a part of the department of Clinical
Pharmacology at University College Hospital Medical
school had done some work in 1979 on the effect
selenium had on cancer. But in 1982 experimental work
on rats and mice was carried out – work which led to
enthusiastic and optimistic hopes that the role of selenium
in reducing tumours had been taken a stage further.
Animals were given carcinogenic agents and at the same
time were given selenium either in the diet or in their
drinking water. The incidence of cancer was found to be
inversely proportional to the concentration of selenium
that was given. In one trial the incidence of tumours in 12
months old mice was reduced from 82 per cent to 48 per
cent in a group given two parts selenium per million and
to 12 per cent in another group given selenium in three
times the strength. Further experiments showed reduced
tumours in animals having less selenium. In another
experiment selenium given to rats was shown to reduce
the total number of tumours of the colon.

The trials concluded that: 'These experiments indicate
that selenium added to the diet inhibits artificially induced
tumours and also spontaneous mammary tumours in
female breeding rats.' The research group referred to the
questions which still needed answering when it came to
selenium but noted the continuing amount of research in
what they called a 'very interesting micronutrient'. There
was a considerable reaction to the London experiments.
In late 1982 one US researcher said that the weight of
informed opinion and research had shown that selenium
was a far from ordinary trace element, and called for

investments into controlled clinical trials. Another spoke at a major New York symposium of the 'excitement' concerning the investigations all over the world into selenium. But it was in California in late 1982 that the strongest voices came for major medical research into selenium and the way it may be influential in the fight against cancer.

A group of doctors whose work had begun at the National Cancer Clinic in Maryland had been lobbying for funds to look into trace elements and their action in the body. In a major presentation they outlined existing research in documented form and said that the onus was on medical research to take deeper steps into the understanding of selenium. And there are signs that clinical trials will begin soon as a result of those pleas. The emphasis is likely to be on developing and adapting Dr Schrauzer's work. As one researcher admitted: 'We have a lot of groundwork to base investigations on. We need to look at the way this particular trace element occurs in the soil and how it can be transformed into the body's system into something that clearly has a considerable effect on cell formulation and the resistance to cancerous growths. We know the more selenium there is in the average diet the less evidence there has been of cancer. That is just the starting point.'

Selenium Intakes World-wide
In Japan, Thailand, the Philippines and other parts of the Far East where blood selenium levels ranged from 0.26 to 0.29 parts per million the breast cancer rate was 0.8 to 8.5 per 100,000. In the United States where blood selenium levels were lower, ranging from 0.07 to 0.20 parts per million, the breast cancer rate was higher, with 19 to 23 people suffering out of 100,000.

In Venezuela, the death rate from cancer of the large intestine was three people out of 100,000. Venezuela has a high selenium content in its soils. Japan, another high-selenium country enjoys a lower lung cancer death rate of 12 people out of 100,000. In the United States, the figure is 37 out of the same number – over three times higher – and the United States has a lower selenium intake.

And what of the U.K? Research by Janet Thorn and Jean Robertson and others for the Ministry of Agriculture Fisheries and Food showed in 1977 that the total intake and amounts of selenium in major foods were low. And they identified they were low because there was a distinct low level of the element in British soil. The publication of their findings at once succeeded in altering the opinions of many people who were unsure of the importance and role of selenium.

Cancer Research
Of the twenty-seven countries studied by Dr Schrauzer and others, the United Kingdom was second only to the Netherlands for the number of instances of death from breast cancer. Twenty-five people out of 100,000 died within the test period. The apparent selenium intake was amongst the lowest recorded. Dr Schrauzer has made no secret of his views. In 1979, he told a special cancer workshop at the National Cancer Institute in Maryland in the United States that the 'key to cancer prevention lies in assuring the adequate intake of selenium as well as other essential trace elements.'

Schrauzer has also said: 'If a breast cancer patient has low selenium levels in her blood, her tendency to develop metastases (other tumours) is increased, her possibility for survival is diminished and her prognosis in general is poorer than if she has normal levels. If every woman started taking selenium today or had a high selenium diet, within a few years the breast cancer rate would drastically decline.' Also in 1979, he spoke at the second International Conference on Inorganic and Nutritional Aspects of Cancer in California and said: 'Selenium supplementation is recommended particularly for individuals at high risk. This includes those with familial predisposition to cancer. Workers in the chemical and metal industries could also benefit from selenium supplementation.'

If there was ever any doubt about the relationship

between cancer deaths and selenium intakes it was probably reduced greatly by a study which looked at various cities within the United States. Generally, the United States is a low-selenium area but as in most countries the glacial action has left some areas with a higher amount of selenium than others. Rapid City in South Dakota has the lowest cancer rate of any city in the United States. The citizens of that city also have the highest measured blood selenium levels. At the other end of the scale in Lima in Ohio which has twice the cancer rate of Rapid City, the blood selenium levels are 60 per cent lower. The full table of results compiled between 1962 and 1966 speak for themselves:

City	Blood Selenium Levels mcg/100ml	Cancer Deaths per 100,000
Rapid City, S.D.	25.6	94.0
Cheyenne, Wyoming	23.4	104.0
Spokane, Washington	23.0	179.0
Fargo, N.D.	21.7	142.0
Little Rock, Ark.	20.1	176.0
Phoenix, Arizona	19.7	126.7
Meridian, Miss.	19.5	125.0
Missoula, Mont.	19.4	174.0
El Paso, Texas	19.2	119.0
Red Bluff, Calif.	18.2	176.0
Geneva, New York	18.2	172.0
Montpelier, Washington	18.0	164.0
Lubbock, Texas	17.8	115.0
Lafayette, L.A.	17.6	145.0
Muncie, Indiana	15.8	169.0
Lima, Ohio	15.7	188.0

Dr Richard Passwater's research into the effects of selenium on cancer led him to believe that the real problem was the deficiency of selenium. It was not just a question of growing concern about the fact that too many people were eating too many fats. 'Fats are not the problem,' he said. 'The problem is that we are eating too many fats for the amount of antioxidants that we get.'

More and more research is now becoming available on selenium, and it continues to highlight the exciting trend. A series of international symposiums in the United States has heard a range of papers presented about the mineral's anti-cancer effect. Drs Clark Griffin and Helen Lane of the University of Texas Health Centre told one meeting that their initial work had been developed and added to. They reported: 'Increasing numbers of chemicals reportedly inhibit or delay the formation of tumours in animals exposed to a variety of cancer-causing agents. Several studies related to the inhibition of chemically induced cancers by administration of selenium compounds have been conducted in our laboratories. The administration of four to five parts per million of selenium in the drinking water or in a form of selenium-enriched yeast added to the diet resulted in a greater than 50 per cent reduction in the number of colon tumours at the end of the study. An extension of this same approach also provided indication that selenium inhibited the induction of tumours in rats given the active hepacarcinogens.' They went on to report that: 'A most important aspect is the possible projection of this approach to prevention of cancer in humans.'

At the same symposium, Mr Milner of Indiana University reported that selenium was seen to be having a noticeable effect on limiting the growth of tumours. 'Recent studies in our laboratory have shown that selenium is capable of retarding the growth of various transplantable tumour cells. The degree of inhibition is dependent upon the form of selenium administered and the quantity given.' He was able to report that tests on mice with tumours showed the selenium slowed the progress of the growth down considerably.

Progress in Selenium Research
A spokesman for the National Cancer Clinic in Maryland

said, perhaps better than anyone else what the progress being made in selenium research meant.

'Through the very considerable work that has been done, not only in this country but at such places as the British Columbia Cancer Research Centre in Canada, in Britain and at some centres in Japan and Germany we feel there is a reason for us to be more confident about the future control of some forms of cancer. We have accepted the premise that selenium can act to protect the body from cancer. In 1956, reports had been submitted which showed that an organic compound called selenocystine, a compound of selenium, had some striking results in the treatment of leukaemia. What has to be remembered is since then over a period of 25 years there has been research by some of the most eminent and respected researchers in the United States. Their work has helped us to build up considerable knowledge. We are not talking now hypothetically about what we hope might be seen in the future.

'We are looking from a position of strength and saying that selenium can become a major line of defence for the body as it fights against cancer. There has very recently been some very important work done with existing cancer patients. There has been a response to treatment. By adding selenium to diets we have seen that there is evidence that the body responds. This is where the major work will develop into [sic]. Is it possible to link a selenium diet with the normal therapy which hospital doctors wish to maintain?

'We have a responsibility to our research programme and that must be our priority, but it is fair to say that we have recorded instances of patients making full recovery from what was considered to be cancer so serious that operations were not thought to be possible. In others, progression of the disease has been stopped.'

The danger is, of course, in all dealings with cancer that sensational reports of a miracle cure will both damage the value of the research work and be treated with vast sceptism by the public. Some criticism has been aimed at the fact that animal experiments are the only ones to have yielded results with selenium. In his book *Cancer and Its Nutritional Therapies*, Dr Richard Passwater says: 'Animal experiments have to be used before human clinical trials can begin. This was seen with the elaborate groundwork required to test vitamin A's protective role in the human bladder cancer. Until human trials are approved, we have to rely on animal studies and test-tube studies using human cell cultures.' He and others know there is a long way to go.

There are many questions still to be answered, but more and more scientists believe that the effect selenium can have on the body is a most exciting and original discovery. The protection it can give to cell membranes and the link it has with vitamin E to work synergistically to stimulate an immune response are beyond doubt. But then there are quite a few other things which are beyond doubt. For instance, the fact that more cancer occurs in areas where there is a low level of selenium in the soil and that adding selenium to the diets of cancer patients has improved their survival time after therapy; the fact that tests show selenium may reduce breast cancer to 80 per cent of its present level and that selenium protects animals that have been fed cancer-causing compounds from succumbing to the disease.

7.

TOWARDS A
HEALTHIER HEART

Let us start in China – with some children... It may seem a bit odd to begin this section by looking at the world's greatest killer – heart disease – not only in China but with Chinese children; but then there is rather a special story to tell.

It concerns a form of heart disease called Keshan's disease, which is a killer. Children and women of child-bearing age are the most susceptible to it. This disease is more common on that huge belt of land running from the north-east to the south-west of China than anywhere else. It is also an area with a very low level of selenium in the soil.

In 1974, a study was made on the effect of selenium on this type of heart disease. It took the form of extra selenium being given to a group of children in Mianning country. Selenium supplements were given to 4,510 children who had been selected at random. Another 3,980 were given the placebo. Twelve months later the numbers in the groups were increased, with 6,709 receiving extra selenium supplements and 5,445 being given the placebo or dummy.

What happened was startling – so dramatic, in fact, that the control group was abolished and all the 13,000 children involved were switched to the selenium. The results had shown themselves to be so successful that no one wanted to give the placebo to any children who might have been at risk. In four communes in the Mianning country, 99 per cent of the children aged one to nine had, in the end, taken part in this remarkable clinical trial. The results literally brought new life to those communes. In 1976, when the selenium was given to all the children there were only four cases of Keshan's disease – a rate of 0.3 per cent. Twelve months after that it was found that there was not one single fresh case in the group of 13,000 children being given the selenium. Yet only two years before that, of the 3,985 children in the original trial group there were 54 cases of the disease – a rate of 1.35 per cent. The death rate in the groups had been cut – and cut drastically.

Dr Gerhard Schrauzer is one of many scientists who have spent a lot of time studying the results. Keshan's disease has now become identified as a selenium deficiency disease. Dr Schrauzer reported: 'Keshan disease does not only occur in Keshan province, but in other parts of central China as well. It turns out that in some very wet regions you can also have a low selenium level. So you can have a leaching out effect there, whereas in the dry parts often you have more selenium. I think in China you just have some parts that are very low in selenium geographically.' The link between the disease and the lack of selenium is powerful. Without selenium there was a major heart disease which was taking lives. By introducing extra selenium into the diet through sodium selenite the disease was controlled and finally eliminated in the children who took part.

There were two extra points; the first was that the Keshan region is not known as a fish eating area and fish is one of the stronger sources of selenium. The second concerns the form in which the selenium was given to the children. For although the trials were very successful, there was a belief that the sodium form used was not the most effective. Dr Schrauzer said: 'They did use sodium selenite and I'm not saying that it's not effective, but they had to use much higher dosages than the recommended allowances. They had to use on the order of a thousand micrograms. That's the drawback. If you use inorganic selenium you have to use very high dosages to get an effect. People who use inorganic selenium must violate their dietary allowances – and that's why I'm against it.'

Before we finish with Keshan's disease, one other study has been of more than a little significance. It concerns a New Zealand patient with a heart disease which had all the infamous features of Keshan's disease. For two years the patient had received intravenous feeding. His condition, which included a paralyzing muscular pain, disappeared after selenium had been given to him through an intravenous solution. It had been thought that symptoms of the disease were consistent with everything which was known about selenium deficiency. Later biochemic findings certainly confirmed that view – there was a marked selenium deficiency.

The Pattern of Heart Disease
It is not stating the case too strongly to say that all the evidence that we now have after years of research supports the fact that if you do not provide your body with enough selenium, you are more likely to get some form of heart disease. It also supports the view that the heart muscles require selenium and we shall see quite clearly that heart disease death rates are much higher in low selenium areas.

But first to the pattern of heart diseases and why they strike. More than 80 per cent of adult heart disease in Western countries is caused by an obstructive disease of the coronary arteries called atherosclerosis. It is derived from the Greek word for porridge, a graphic way of describing the material which builds up in the arteries of the body. When the silting up of the arteries begins, it starts in the form of small, yellow patches or streaks. These patches enlarge, projecting into the arteries until

they eventually start to interfere or even block the blood
flow. The process is a slow one, taking place over a period
of years. The enlarged patches are normally known as
plaques and thought of as deposits of cholesterol. The
plaque which carries the cholesterol actually begins as a
mutated or damaged muscle cell and grows into the
innermost layer of the artery. But the important thing is
that the arteries must remain open to allow adequate
amounts of blood through. When the plaque reaches an
advanced stage, various complications can start to occur.
The surface of the plaque may break down and form a raw
area where a clot may develop. This clotting is called
thrombosis.

There has been an enormous weight of research by
scientists, surgeons, doctors and pathologists into the
causes of such heart diseases. The three most important
are cigarette smoking, high blood pressure and abnormal
blood fats. But there are also other factors which affect
the pattern – factors such as stress, a family history of
heart disease, lack of exercise and being overweight. One
important distinguishing factor is being a member of the
male sex. Men are twice as likely to be hit by heart disease
as women.

Country	Heart Disease Rate	Selenium Intake
Finland	1009	25
U.S.A.	870	61
Canada	722	62
Ireland	722	75
Great Britain	713	75
Australia	867	76
Norway	602	82
Greece	236	92
Poland	301	94
Yugoslavia	232	99
Bulgaria	331	108

*The research featured heart disease deaths per 100,000 in
55 to 64 year-old men.*

Selenium's Role in Heart Disease

Take a look at the following figures. They show the rate of coronary heart disease in countries throughout the world. Alongside them the estimated daily intake of selenium (in micrograms) is shown.

The single most dramatic results with selenium have come recently from research based at the Cleveland Clinic in the United States where reports were collated from 24 countries looking at heart disease and selenium content of the respective soils. There, results showed that Finland and the United States which are known to have some of the world's lowest selenium levels have four to five times more instances of heart attacks than countries such as Yugoslavia where the selenium content is one of the highest in the world.

Another study conducted by a Finnish doctor, Johan A. Bjorksten, found that heart attacks are three or four times more common in countries with 0.05 parts per million of selenium in water supplies than in countries with 0.10 parts per million. The amounts are minutely different; the effect such small amounts have on the quality of life are quite staggering. In the population between the working ages of 15 and 64, he noted that heart attacks are seven times more prevalent in the low-selenium areas. In early 1981, a study within Finland showed that variations of selenium levels within the country directly related to the amount of recorded heart diseases in certain areas.

In 1973, the World Health Organization included selenium among the five elements which it thought needed to be studied in relation to coronary heart disease. Since then more and more studies in China, Finland, New Zealand, the United States and Great Britain have been carried out and have shown that there is a direct link between selenium deficiency and heart diseases.

Early studies with this mineral had convinced animal nutritionists that selenium deficiencies were the cause of nutritional muscular dystrophy. The role of selenium as an antioxidant suggested that there might be a case for investigating the effect the trace mineral might have on the formation of plaque in the arteries. Research became aimed towards the theory that the free radicals harmed the cells which were fighting back by pulling cholesterol out of the blood stream. More and more researchers in the 1970's published their studies linking selenium deficiencies in various animals to heart disease.

In 1968, the United States Department of Agriculture told chicken and turkey farmers to put selenium concentrations into their animal feed or to inject animals with selenium soon after birth. That advice followed research by Dr Milton Scott that selenium-deficient chickens and turkeys quickly developed heart degeneration. The loss of animals through disease was a serious financial threat to farmers and they had to take action to put things right. This became a major concern. The poultry was the first to be identified since half the number of chickens and turkeys were being raised in selenium-deficient areas and were causing annual losses of millions of dollars.

But poultry was not the only problem. It was likely to have an effect on cattle, sheep, pigs and goats. In 1973, Canada approved the addition of selenium to poultry and swine feeds. Twelve months later, the United States Department of Agriculture followed suit. It issued document AT 15768 which noted the importance of selenium in healthy animals, and pointed out that vast areas of the United States were not able to provide enough selenium from natural sources.

If the shortage had produced a scare for animals then the need to apply the research and findings to human beings became critical. A Soviet research team discovered that selenium was needed to minimize the damage caused by heart attacks. They blocked the flow of blood in a coronary artery and measured the extent of the damage. Extra selenium was found to decrease the extent of heart damage. Time and again, it seemed that selenium was acting as a protector for the cell membranes. The presence of free radicals meant that cells in the body were spreading just as in cancer. They were out of control and causing deposits in the arteries of the heart.

Dr Richard Passwater links selenium to the operation of coenzyme Q. This coenzyme – also called ubiquinone – is an aid to certain reactions in the body which help the heart to function better. Dr Passwater says: 'Since the normal human heart is higher in coenzyme Q content than most other tissues it follows that biopsy samples taken from the hearts of heart disease patients show a deficiency of coenzyme Q. Animal studies have shown that a deficiency of coenzyme Q lessens heart vitality and produces cardiac degenerative lesions. Selenium appears to be the most important nutrient in the control of its levels. Therefore, adequate selenium is required to produce the necessary coenzyme Q required for a healthy heart.'

We have seen throughout this book that selenium makes things happen in the body. It is known to be able to detoxify trace metal poisons that enter the body. Cadmium, for example, is an atmospheric pollutant in many industrial cities and its accumulation in the kidneys is believed to cause cases of hypertension and high blood pressure. Selenium can break down such cadmium build-ups.

Throughout the ever-increasing research programme, one single fact seems to be more relevant and more important than any other. That is that fewer people die from heart diseases in places where there is enough selenium in the soil. We have seen that in one area of China a killer heart disease was virtually wiped out by providing communes with 1000 micrograms of selenium each week. This is not the end of the story. Three-year clinical trials have started in Finland, linking the use of selenium with vitamin E, and the need of success is urgent since far more people die of heart-related diseases in Scandinavia than anywhere else in the world. As one of the research team said: 'The world needs these trials to be positive and to build up this evidence. But we in Finland perhaps need it most.'

8.

VITAMIN E AND SELENIUM –
A GREAT DOUBLE ACT

Vitamin E is a bit like a bodyguard. One of the most important things it does is protect essential nutrients such as vitamin A, vitamin C, amino acids and polyunsaturated fatty acids. It acts as an antioxidant in preventing these substances being broken down and losing their strength, both in the food we eat and in the body itself.

But if vitamin E is the bodyguard, then selenium is the 'tough guy' or 'right-hand man'. Together they form quite a team. Research has now established that the two nutrients work synergistically – they have a greater effect working together than they do separately; and it is no coincidence that research work into both vitamin E and selenium has time and again overlapped until it became obvious that there was a strong and powerful link between the two.

Vitamin E has been labelled recently as the 'vitality vitamin'. It can keep you looking younger by retarding the ageing of cells from oxidation, aid the heart by preventing and dissolving blood clots, act as a diuretic and lower blood pressure. It can also act as a protective agent against pollution. A deficiency in this vitamin, the best natural sources of which are vegetable oils, wheat germ, wholemeal bread, egg yolks, green vegetables, and nuts, can often cause muscular disorders. So straight away we can see that the way vitamin E has been identified as helping the body can be directly linked and associated with the sort of benefits found from selenium.

The Fight Against the 'Baddies'
When we looked at the effect selenium may have on cancer, ageing and heart disease there was a phrase which kept cropping up. It was 'free radicals' - and it is the way vitamin E and selenium work to attack these free radicals or 'baddies' that holds the key to their joint function. We have seen already that the human body contains an almost incalculable number of cells. There may be over 60,000,000,000 000 (60 trillion) of them and they are all the time under attack from free radicals which are highly reactive fragments of molecules which can cause chain reaction damage.

What happens is that these fragments link up with, and get extra strength from, the fatty constituents of the cell and they multiply. It is this oxidization of the cell which has now become linked with diseases of many parts of the body. Vitamin E, vitamin C and selenium provide the body with the ability to fight back. They are three strong antioxidants and by far the most powerful one is selenium.

Dr Doug Frost, researcher at the Trace Mineral Laboratory in New York has spent much time looking at the way selenium and Vitamin E work together. He has said that: 'There is a unique relationship between vitamin E and selenium which will have wide-ranging benefits to health and the extension of useful lifespan. We now know so much more about the way they can work to reduce oxidative damage and damage from heavy metals. Opportunities for prevention or curative applications of selenium, combined with E and other essential nutrients, seem compelling and warrant attention in clinical nutrition and medicine.'

The way they work in the body synergistically is believed to be concentrated in an enzyme, or part of one specific enzyme by the name of glutathione peroxidase. Enzymes speed up the body's reactions – they keep everything in top gear and functioning properly. Glutathione peroxidase is a protective enzyme which will not work properly without selenium and vitamin E.

More and more is being found out about the way these two nutrients team up. Clinical trials have been held in Mexico where nine out of ten patients suffering from angina who were treated with vitamin E and selenium found a reduction in the number of attacks. In this instance, the two nutrients were used together in a drug called tolsem. There was no evidence of side effects with the treatment. Two other major investigations have been carried out, specifically looking at the way vitamin E and selenium work together. Soviet researcher Dr T. Berenshtein found that supplements of selenium plus vitamin E produced more antibodies to help the body resist infection from bacteria and viruses. Selenium itself had very little effect, and there was none at all with vitamin E. But together the results were remarkable.

Another recent test was concerned with giving selenium to cancer patients, in a dosage of up to 2000 micrograms daily – ten times over any sort of recommended dose – along with other antioxidants including the vitamins A, C, and E. The doctor would adjust the selenium supplementation to produce normal blood selenium levels which often did not occur until 900 to 2000 micrograms were given every day. After that he found no evidence of nerve, liver or blood abnormalities.

The weight of the research is now formidable. Twelve centres in the world have entered into a second more complex programme after obtaining encouraging results from their initial work with selenium and vitamin E. Clinical trials are also under way. The theory being developed is that vitamin E may have stolen some of the glory it did not deserve; and the vitamin may be covering for a problem in selenium deficiency. There is also scope for the theory that if vitamin E fails to be beneficial in some areas, it may be because it does not have the help of its 'right-hand man' - selenium. It may be equally true that selenium enhances the vitamin's action.

Vitamin E and Selenium Against Muscular Dystrophy

Much of the work into muscular dystrophy has focussed on vitamin E. In the absence of any drugs to correct the condition, many doctors have sought a correction of the cause rather than the condition itself. They have used vitamin E in large doses - and found it has slowed down the development of the disease. The tragedy of muscular dystrophy is that it is a progressive disease whose characteristic is a wasting away of stripped muscles in the body. The muscles degenerate and are replaced by fat or fibrous tissues. Most commonly affected are the shoulder muscles together with those of the face, the muscles at the back of the thighs and the calf muscles. As a disease, it often strikes between the ages of two and five.

Vitamin E was thought to hold much promise by using it in such doses as to either rejuvenate cells or just to allow the human body to absorb fat - the major source of vitamin E. The research was concentrated on animals and attempts to link what was happening with vitamin E in the treatment of animals with what it might do to aid human beings proved to be very difficult. As long ago as 1962 a university group demonstrated that selenium and vitamin E could prevent muscular dystrophy in lambs. A five-year research programme, including feeding selenium-and-vitamin E-low foodstuffs showed that muscular disorders became more common. When both nutrients were given to the ewes, the dystrophy was wiped out. There have been other successful tests on animals which led to veterinarians using the combinations as a treatment.

But is the same action likely to be true for humans? Some suggested links to vitamin E have also been discounted. That has led to the belief that there is an unbreachable difference between animal and human dystrophies. One link may be coenzyme Q - or ubiquinone which, as we have seen in the way selenium acts on heart problems, is an aid in certain reactions in the body, reactions which have helped to strengthen the heart. This particular coenzyme has successfully been tried out on monkeys suffering from muscular dystrophy. Selenium is needed for the production of it and there has been a call to develop the initial thinking that vitamin E may have a role to play in aiding muscular dystrophy to include selenium.

The roles of the two nutrients have come to be accepted now as being interchangeable. The work of Dr Denman Harman, president of the American Ageing Association, has been crucial. He has shown that vitamin E and antioxidants extended the average life expectancy of mice. He extensively researched the role of free radicals in the ageing process and was able to conclude that diets aimed at cutting back such reactions 'may reasonably be expected to add five to ten or more years of healthy productive life to the lifespan of the average person'. He had highlighted very powerfully the importance of these two nutrients in the diet.

9.

SELENIUM IN OUR FOOD

There is now widespread conviction that selenium is a vital trace element and that we need it in our bodies. The trouble is that we can aim to eat more of the right sort of foods in an attempt to get more selenium, only to find there is not enough in the soil to give us as much as we need. The major research by the Ministry of Agriculture, Fisheries and Food, undertaken by Janet Thorn and Jean Robertson, produced a few very worrying statistics.

What they found was that the total intake and amounts of selenium in major foods were low because there was such a poor level of the element in British soil. And research into those levels shows that only in North Norfolk are there adequate amounts to ensure that crops grown in the selenium-rich soil can provide us with the amount we need. Some areas of Devon and others in Southern Ireland are marginally higher than the rest of the U.K., but even they are not quite high enough.

The best sources of selenium are those where other trace minerals are found – cereals, nuts, vegetables, fruits, seafoods and the organ meats. In vegetables, the amounts are very small, among the exceptions are asparagus and garlic, but not many people are too eager to eat either of those in abundance. Over-cooking can also reduce the selenium content of foods. The selenium compounds are very volatile. Heat, processing and cooking can drastically affect the content. The refining of wheat can destroy about half to three-quarters of the total selenium content of the whole grain. Boiling may cut about 45 per cent of the selenium content. White flour and white bread production has been known to lose 80 per cent.

One estimate claims that a well balanced diet can, in the U.K., provide between 60 and 80 micrograms of selenium. (The average is 60 micrograms.) The sort of recommended daily intake now being suggested is between 100 and 200 micrograms. So, even eating the right things, prepared in the right way, is not going to be good enough to reach the level of intake which doctors suggest. Ministry of Agriculture figures in 1978 said that half of the average selenium intake in this country came from cereals and cereal products. Forty per cent came from fish and meat together. So how much selenium do you think you are getting?

Take a quick look at the following relative food levels of selenium. They will give you a guide to show which type of foods are selenium-rich. Many such food tables can give false impressions, because one area and its selenium content can vary enough to alter the amount processed through the food grown in its soil. This table is meant to show you how the values of different foods compare.

Nutritionists have become concerned about selenium taken into the body through food because it is not just a question of not getting the right quantities. Much of the selenium which is contained in the food we eat comes in a form which is poorly absorbed or utilized by the body. The crucial factor is not how much of this mineral we eat, but how much of it passes into the cells of the body. One particular worry is that many turn to fish and say that a fish diet can overcome any deficiency. Unfortunately,

Food	Selenium (mg) per 100g
Bread	0.002
Cereal products	0.019
Broad beans	0.003
Other beans	0.004
Eggs	0.021
Vegetables	0.004
Fruits	0.003
Meat	0.014
Fish	0.016
Poultry	0.013
Milk	0.001
Cheese	0.001
Sugar	0.0

much of the selenium in the fish is bound to mercury and cannot be absorbed.

The concern at this lack of absorption is summed up in tests prepared for teenagers in the United States, which deal with balanced diets, thought to provide adequate selenium. The food was carefully selected and prepared. The analysis was done by an accurate activation system. And in one of the tests, five sample diets were without any trace of selenium.

The Missing Element in the Soil
Several leading figures in the nutrition field in Britain had been hovering on the brink of a significant discovery for quite a while. The evidence about selenium was building up all the time, but were the experts really convinced of its crucial role? The single piece of evidence which persuaded most people was the report in 1977 which underlined the fact that Britain's soil was very low in selenium content.

Heavily populated areas in the Midlands and North were some of the worst areas, but for Britain as a whole it was a poor picture. The distribution of selenium in the soil varies greatly throughout the world. For the most part, areas which have been glaciated in the prehistoric past tend to be those with the lowest selenium levels. The United States, Canada, New Zealand and areas of Europe such as Scandinavia and Great Britain are the worst hit, but even in areas where the selenium content is fairly high now, the soil is being stripped of this valuable trace element because of modern fertilization practices and acid rain.

At the heart of the problem is the sulphur-rich artificial fertilizers, known to inhibit the intake of selenium by plants and vegetables. Levels of sulphur in the soil are being raised annually, and in such amounts which are slowly but surely wearing down the existing levels of selenium. Deficiency of the mineral became a very real problem for the sheep industry in some parts of the United States – but only after the high sulphur content fertilizers started to be used.

Other factors which are lowering the concentration of selenium in the soil include the removal of this substance by crops and the fact that most of the selenium from oil and coal burning ends up in a form which cannot join the food process and be taken up by plants. All of which results in the sort of claim made by Dr Douglas Frost that pollution, soil deterioration and modern fertilizers had 'greatly inhibited the uptake of selenium by plants'. And he added: 'Evidence suggests that diminished selenium availability may be worldwide.'

Dr Richard Passwater takes up the claim that something should be done to redress the balance. But is this possible? Unless we fertilize soils or supplement animal feeds with selenium we will find it impractical, if not next to impossible, to obtain optimal levels of selenium. Until selenium supplementation of all animal feeds is permitted farmers should be encouraged to use selenium and vitamin E injections to make their livestock and their customers healthy.

'Fertilization is more difficult, however. Some crops cannot grow if too much selenium is applied to the soil

while other plants can concentrate selenium to a degree
which could be toxic to livestock. Fertilization of alkaline
soils with selenium produces oxidation products that are
readily soluble and washed away. Fertilization of acid
soils with selenium may result in poor selenium uptake.'

So it seems that man can no longer rely on nature for
supplies of selenium. In too many countries there simply
is not enough of it. In others, it is being eradicated and
supplies are fading away with limited chances of them
being replenished.

How Much Selenium Do We Need?

One of the hardest things to come to terms with involving
this quite remarkable trace mineral is that when we talk
about how much the body needs we are talking in
quantities as small as a millionth of a gram – or micrograms.
The story of this book is concerned with man's increasing
problem in providing enough selenium for the needs of
his body.

But how much do we need? Too little will not allow the
element to perform its health-giving functions; too much
is thought to have its own dangers. The recent Ministry of
Agriculture, Fisheries and Food report suggested that
while the average daily intake in Britain was only 60
micrograms, there was a basic need for all of us to have an
intake of something between 80 and 200 micrograms.
The trouble with the official 'Ministry view' is that it
leaves a lot of scope between the two figures. So, both in
the United States and in Britain, a tentative figure of 150
micrograms per day has been suggested. That figure has
to be viewed in the knowledge that the average 'good
diet' will provide between 35 and 60 micrograms a day. In
Britain, you can only reach a level of 150 micrograms as a
daily intake by eating selenium-rich foods in a high
selenium area. The problem is that there is only one tiny
area where such a situation could develop.

It is probably worth looking at the opinions of two
leading researchers into the effects of selenium, namely,
Drs Schrauzer and Shamberger who both agree that a

daily adult selenium intake should be as high as 250 to 350 micrograms a day. Their joint thinking is that dietary estimates were based on more selenium being available twenty or thirty years ago than there is today. The selenium has been eroded, so therefore much less is present in our food; and therefore the experts believe that people do not eat as well or as sensibly as nutritionists like to think. What seems to be a typical diet to a nutritionist is only an occasional diet to the average person. It is also worth noting that Japanese fishermen eating large amounts of selenium-rich fish have been calculated to exceed 500 micrograms of the mineral every day – with no harmful effect.

When selenium supplements first became available in health food stores in the United States, the controlling Food and Drug Administration tried to ban them, claiming that selenium was not a nutrient but an untested food additive. The manufacturers and distributors of selenium supplements contested the action – and won the day. Their campaign highlighted the need for and safety of supplements containing selenium. In a letter of approval the F.D.A. said that it would not take legal action as long as the recommended daily dose did not exceed 200 micrograms. It was that view which led to the strengthening of a compromise; the selenium-rich foods were said to be of value in the provision of selenium, but it was decided that extra selenium should be taken as a supplement.

Can You Take Too Much Selenium?
The answer is simple. You can – but it would be very difficult to do so. Anything up to 1100 micrograms of selenium a day is said to be a safe level – and that is ten times what is being recommended to us. In fact, clinical trials on adults who consumed 2000 micrograms daily for periods over a month have failed to show any signs of toxicity. So while it is as well to be aware of the toxic limit of the mineral, there is very little reason to be concerned. All minerals can be toxic and there is no reason to fear it for that alone.

There is no danger that diet will provide an excess of selenium. As we have seen, Japanese fishermen who literally live on fish all day and every day, are a long way from displaying any toxicity level. The only danger is in taking too much supplementation and since stated doses and courses are clearly marked on the products available on the market, there is no need for concern.

Selenium Supplements

Like other trace elements, selenium is better absorbed by the body in an organic form. Yeast grown in the presence of selenium, so that the mineral is incorporated into the yeast cell itself, is the safest and the most efficient way to take selenium. The breakthrough for this particular method came in 1974 when a type of brewer's yeast was developed in which selenium was bound to the protein part of the yeast cell. The advantages are that the selenium yeast is biologically formed and is one third as toxic as the inorganic selenium in the form of sodium selenite. Quite stringent tests on this particular form and its toxicity have been carried out and found to be safe. The selenium yeast has been tested for biological efficacy, both on human beings and animals. It is absorbed into the body and made to work on the action of the cells ten to twenty times more efficiently than the organic product.

Organic materials are usually better absorbed into the body because they are chelated. In the chelation process, the mineral is surrounded by amino acids and a complex reaction occurs. Selenium has different characteristics and does not undergo the same process.

Selenium researchers have carried out tests on supplements on the market – and have passed them as being safe and effective. They recommend the organic form and know more about selenium yeast than the other forms now being looked at. So it makes sense to make use of their knowledge and experience. The progress of selenium supplements was, for a while, held up by toxicity fears. Those fears have now been eliminated and perfectly safe forms of the mineral are now available, some of them taking advantage of the synergistic way it can work with vitamin E and the known benefits of taking in vitamins A and C, all powerful antioxidants.

10.

WHAT OF THE FUTURE?

Ten years ago, few people would have dared predict the development in our knowledge and understanding of the role of selenium. The idea that selenium and vitamin E both protected the body's cells from breakdown hinted that they might be crucial to many functions.

Although the picture is far from complete, we still have a much clearer idea of the details surrounding selenium's contribution to our health. Selenium is not a panacea, a cure for everything and anything. It has specific and identifiable functions in the body. There may be findings in the future which will spread new light on some of the evidence we have been looking at.

Selenium Against Cystic Fibrosis
There is an increasing call, for instance, to develop the way selenium can act as a protection against cystic fibrosis, the disease which can clog the lungs and digestive system. The vast majority of researchers believe that cystic fibrosis is caused by a genetic effect. Dr Joel Wallach has suggested that it may be due to a selenium

deficiency. He has examined children suffering from the disease and found very low selenium levels. In a survey of 15 mothers with cystic fibrosis children, he found that many of the pregnancies and deliveries were both stormy and complicated. There were ten miscarriages. Eight pregnancies resulted in significant hair loss or change in hair character-features associated with selenium and zinc deficiencies in laboratory animals. Also, there is the fact that cystic fibrosis occurs more frequently in low selenium areas in the United States.

Dr Wallach has developed a treatment which has been successful. He recommends that cystic fibrosis patients should improve their nutrition by eating a green salad daily, lean meats and liver four times a week, eggs for breakfast daily, cut out wheat and substitute rice and potatoes. He also adds that it is vital to take dietary supplements of selenium, zinc, copper and vitamin E. It is a therapy which has received a lot of publicity – basically because it has had some startling results. Dr Wallach adds: 'The natural history and patient profile of the predominantly perinatal disease complex known as cystic fibrosis fits that of an acquired environmental disease that can be produced by a deficiency of selenium, zinc and riboflavin and can be aggravated and precipitated by a low vitamin E diet that is rich in polyunsaturated fatty acids.'

The Children's Lung Association in the United States has taken up the lead and has also had excellent results. Dr Roy Goddard, president of the association, has been quoted as saying he thought it was one of the biggest breakthroughs since the discovery of the disease. He said that twelve patients on a special diet of foods rich in trace elements plus extra supplements of selenium, zinc and copper had made considerable progress.

General Resistance to Disease
Research in the future may unlock a few more doors in the bid to discover what other benefits selenium might have. Three independent trials began in the summer of 1981 to look at the broader implications selenium may

hold for the future. Its relationship with vitamin E is well known – but what other trace elements would it work with? There is a possibility that selenium may be able to increase the body's general resistance to disease and this is now the subject of trials in the United States. Selenium may also be found to improve resistance to many diseases caused by viruses or bacteria. The mineral has certainly been seen to improve the immune response in several animals. Such is the elusiveness of selenium that it may well have a fundamental role to play in the body's in-built defence mechanism against everything from a common cold to tropical diseases. In fact, so much research is now being carried out in these subjects that selenium is one of the most talked about minerals there is. If the next five years are able to reveal to doctors, researchers and nutritionists the same sort of data that has been produced over the past five years then the value of selenium will enter a new phase.

Perhaps it is right that some of the last words should go to two men who have spent so much of their time studying trace minerals. One is Dr David Davies of the Gerontological Unit of University Hospital, London, who says: 'Selenium is a must with the vast increase in the mass production of food for human consumption. Much of the value of these foods is depleted in the processing of plastic foods that go to make up the diet of people in the so-called civilized world. Many other valuable trace elements disappear in the process, natural selenium being one of the first casualties.'

And the other is Dr Richard Passwater who has been researching selenium for the past twenty years. He has said: 'If you want to maintain your health, increase your resistance to disease and assure a long and energetic life it is vitally important that you increase your daily intake of selenium. Unfortunately, most people today are not getting enough of this essential mineral. It doesn't promise to cure whatever ails you. You should not entertain false hopes of a cure just because the evidence suggests that selenium can prevent or alleviate a certain

disease. At the very least you should be aware of the
important roles played by selenium and then optimize
your diet accordingly.'

Selenium and the Birth Rate

The United States National Centre for Health Statistics
and Population Data is, as you might expect, a building
full of facts and figures. In amongst its archives is possibly
one of the most remarkable ones – linking high birth rates
in the United States to areas rich in selenium. It is a
consistent pattern that has been tested critically. A
Pittsburgh University study into the facts states clearly
that 'the high-selenium regions exhibit a higher birth rate
than the medium- and low-selenium areas.'

It proved to be a fascinating and revealing exercise. But
then it is already known that selenium almost certainly
plays a part in the reproductive system. Animals deficient
of the trace mineral fail to reproduce. Selenium is one of
the ingredients of semen in men with sperm cells containing
relatively high amounts. Half of a man's body selenium is
concentrated in the testicles and the seminal glands
which are near the prostate gland. Thus, significant
amounts may be lost in sexual intercourse.

The fact that poor diet has an effect on human reproductive ability is not new. Several research findings have
linked the way selenium and vitamin E work together in
this area and selenium added to the diet of sheep has been
shown to improve the number of births.

The Fight Against Pollution

Do you know what happens when you breathe in fumes
from car exhausts? Well, it is more than likely that you
are exposing your system to cadmium – and to the chance
of heavy metal poisoning. Sophisticated twentieth century
life still succeeds in polluting the air, and cadmium, lead,
arsenic and mercury are all harmful types of minerals.
They are what are known as the heavy metal pollutants
and chronic poisoning can cause sickness in various

forms, ranging from sickness, constipation, severe stomach-ache and fatigue. Cadmium is one of the worst of these offenders. It can come from tobacco smoke as well as from diesel fumes.

However, there is some good news; for selenium is known to be of great use against such metals, and can help to remove them from the system. Equally, a selenium deficiency results in a danger of there being no process in the body to detoxify the minerals. These then build up gradually until their effect is felt. Selenium has a high affinity for these toxic metals, binding on to them and rendering them harmless. It seems to be able to alter the tissue disposition of a number of these metals.

The threat of such poisoning is quite real; cadmium and its resulting high blood pressure is the worst – particularly for smokers. Mercury is more likely to affect health, either through industrial pollution or the remains of pesticides, and arsenic can also enter the body via pesticides or accidental pollution of spices.

Several nutrients are known to help the body fight against these metals, but research at the Trace Mineral Laboratory in New York found that although zinc and some chelating agents are effective in removing cadmium from the body, selenium is by far the most effective. In one test, it was shown to be 100 times as effective as zinc.

The Danger of Radiation

Radiation belongs to that category of words which normally is more suited to a nightmare than anything else. It conjures up a picture of nuclear war and destruction. Yet the accident at the nuclear energy plant on Three Mile Island near Harrisberg, Pennsylvania awakened many fears of the dangers of unexpected radiation. But there are other dangers; dangers from medical treatment such as X-ray, isotope screening and cobalt therapy. In the early 1970's, research substantiated that natural selenium amino acid and protein compounds are tremendous protectors against radiation.

The Latest Developments

Early in 1982 researchers from literally every continent in the world began to pull together the threads of extra knowledge which have recently been discovered about selenium. The focal point of their attention was another in a series of special seminars – this time in Iceland – to update what is known of the effects of this trace element.

In the build-up to the seminar, tests and trials were carried out in Japan, the United States, New Zealand, Finland, West Germany and Canada. A whole series of papers were prepared showing that selenium was not something that was going to be forgotten but rather something that had a much deeper and significant effect on the future health of the human body.

In Japan there has been a lot of research into heart diseases, and in 1981 Kyoto Medical University carried out tests and trials on a group of trace elements and the connection they had with the structure and function of cells. Their success with a whole series of tests on mice and rats, and the effect selenium can have, has led them to begin work on a two year trial using selenium and vitamin E. It will be one of the largest and most significant trials ever carried out and will follow the lines of the trial conducted in Mexico on the drug tolsem (chromalloy). The combination then was said to have demonstrated beneficial effects in 92 per cent of people suffering with heart problems.

In Kyoto there has also been work done on the way selenium can affect the role of free radicals in heart disease. In a recent series of lectures to pharmacists in Japan Dr Taranabe said: 'There is growing evidence to suggest that the more we look into the effects that selenium has the more we shall be able to benefit the day to day ability of the body to combat a number of diseases and illnesses. It is showing itself to be a truly remarkable element. What is important is to be aware of it and learn about it.'

There is little doubt among many leading researchers that selenium can and does have a key part to play in the ageing process, but it has only been in the last three or four years that lengthy experiments have been carried out. And it is only now that the switch has been made from laboratory tests on small animals to humans. If positive results are found in mice and rats then they may well apply to humans – and that has been a gap in the research. Details of a new series of trials using selenium to test the anti-oxidant powers it has to slow down the rate of cell destruction were due to be announced in early 1982.

In the United States at least five trials and tests using selenium were in progress during late 1981. Most of the work done in California, Texas and New York was again due to be presented by research scientists at the international symposium.

In the U.K. the Ministry of Agriculture are set to update their research work during 1982 with a five year follow on which will use as a basis the work done in 1977 which established that selenium levels in Britain were below the minimum requirements being recommended. A spokesman said that the research work which would be done would form part of the package needed to fill gaps in the knowledge of soil contents.

'We are aware of the amount of research work that is going on into trace elements, and in particular selenium. We will be developing our studies in this area along with nutrition needs. The whole area of research is providing us with new channels to investigate which perhaps have been either ignored or just not known about. The research work in 1977 was only the first phase. We believe it is a study that has to continue.'

One of the men to bridge the gap between research on small mammals and tests on humans is Dr Gerhard Schrauzer. In the latest study, selenium yeast was administered at levels of 150 micrograms per day for six weeks. The results showed conclusively that blood selenium levels showed a significant increase – from 0.12 to 0.22. The supplementation experiments were carried out primarily to show that selenium yeast was the most efficient way for humans to absorb the selenium. The next phase was to test the cell formation over a longer period of time.

Indeed most of the crucial second phase work now being carried out by Dr Schrauzer and many others is into the key area of cell formation. Work at Utah University and the United States National Institute of Health is now concentrating on the free radical theory. In the autumn of 1981 a report from the Weizmann Institute of Science endorsed the theory that some organic compounds have a key role to play in the very subtle and complex reactions of cell formation.

'A certain number of free radicals produced when radiation manages to break through to penetrate a cell are now known to be highly reactive. They enter chemical reactions with the chromosomes of the cell and break the chromosomes, destroying some of the information carried by them. The destroyed information may range over any part of the genetic message but sometimes it is that which controls the replication of the cell.'

The next phase was the introduction of a series of organic compounds, primarily selenium, which helped to slow down the damaging process. So, these highly reactive fragments of molecules which spark off a chain reaction, and in turn damage the millions of cells in the body, can be controlled. This has a whole range of implications from the ability of the heart to fight disease to slowing down the ageing process and including the research into muscular dystrophy.

As we have seen, the work being done on this remarkable trace element is not likely to be short-lived. One leading researcher has said that the work of the past ten years has only scratched the surface of what we know or understand about the way minute traces of a mineral can affect the general health and vitality of the body. Late in 1981 a report to the World Health Organization, which itself isolated selenium as one of the key elements worthy of further investigation, stated that the discoveries made into the trace mineral was the 'single most important parcel of work done on natural compounds and man's understanding of them'.

It went on to call for a greater need to speed up research work adding: 'From a very low base of knowledge on selenium ten years ago there has been a large number of laboratory controlled tests and analyses which have shown that the trace element selenium has a key role to play over the next thirty years in the way we control our health. It has been shown to be beneficial in building a healthy heart, and much of the most exciting work has been done in the field of the nutritional therapies towards fighting cancer. The W.H.O. cannot and should not ignore this very exciting work'.

In the autumn of 1981 three men – two of them Japanese and the third from New Zealand – began a series of tests on selenium which took the research into the element into a new era. Their work at Osaka University and other centres in Japan has made use of highly sophisticated instruments which have quite literally helped one aspect of research to change gear. The work, led by Dr Wanaka, has been looking behind the effects of ageing, and specifically at the reason and merits of protein missynthesis. Over the past few years the importance of protein missynthesis – where proteins are not integrated into cells but start a decaying process – has become a controversial issue.

The role of this protein action in the body is complex. As malformed protein increases, an increasing number of cells which need to be regenerated, function poorly and die. Research into this aspect of ageing has been hampered by the difficulty of not being able to record in the laboratory the increase of an almost unlimited kind of missynthesized protein. But in Japan chemical technicians believe they can now delve further into the role of this part of the ageing process. Selenium has been isolated as the best antioxidant and will be used in the tests to show how the possible mechanisms of production of missynthesized proteins can be altered and controlled.

The story of selenium does not end here. What

knowledge has been uncovered in the past twenty years has identified a very remarkable aspect of the role of trace elements. The success story of the benefits of selenium has spread. One researcher has said that it is likely in the late 1980's to be one of the most keenly investigated areas of nutrition.

Almost every month there is some facet of its ability that is uncovered. In the United States the success story has spread from the laboratory through the media to the public who have been made aware of the need to add this important mineral to their diet. In the U.K. the pattern is the same. It has become one of the best 'news stories' in the world of nutrition.

11.

'THANK YOU
FOR HELPING ME'

When *Here's Health* magazine offered its readers the chance to try selenium the response was overwhelming. Of the large number of people who tried it eight out of ten said selenium had brought significant changes to their health. They responded to a special questionnaire and detailed how the product had helped them. Under the general heading 'Thank You for Helping Me' the following is a selection of some of the comments that the magazine received.

General Health
'I have found my stamina has improved beyond all reacognition since I started taking the selenium. I am waking up a lot earlier and I seem to be able to cope a lot more with day to day problems.'

*   *   *

'I found great improvement in the way I coped with the 'daily grind' and I seemed to have got more on an even keel. I have been more alert and seem to fight off colds a lot whereas in the past I was the first person to catch a cold!

*   *   *

'I feel so fit in the mornings now. I dreaded getting up, now I feel better with my nerves. I am enjoying my chores and everything I do.'

*   *   *

'I am more resistant to illnesses and my wife says that I seem so much brighter. I feel that I don't need to have so much sleep and I never get that weary feeling. I don't even fall asleep on the train coming home – I do some work. It has made a big difference to the way I feel. I think my labrador dog is much healthier. I even give the selenium tablets to him. He's 11 years old and has never looked so well and fit. Thanks from both of us.'

Migraine
'I'm very pleased with the product. My migraines are now very infrequent and I'm sure it is all due to taking the selenium. It's too much of a co-incidence.

*   *   *

'Generally I've felt so much more energetic since I started taking the selenium. Migraine has always been one of my worst problems. I'm 61 and I've accepted them. Now I hardly get them at all. They're now so infrequent that I'm able to be quite sure that the selenium has had the effect I hoped it would.'

*   *   *

'Every few days I seemed to get the spots in front of my eyes and the dizzy feeling that I always knew was the start of an attack of migraine. I wasn't taking any prescribed medicines but I took the selenium to see if it would do anything for me. I read a magazine article which said that it had helped with migraine. I have been taking it now for six weeks and it has done me wonderfully. The attacks of migraine have almost disappeared and I feel so much better.'

Nervous problems
'I've always felt very tense and have had a lot of nervous trouble which often seemed to result in stress and trouble. I went through weeks when I couldn't face up to things properly. It gave me a lot of problems at work. I started taking selenium because I do believe in the value of supplements. I have to say that I am a new person in terms of confidence. I don't get nerves any more and I think all my friends see it in me. Selenium works.'

*   *   *

'I'd like to thank you for the selenium. It has had a marked effect on me. I'm no longer nervous or over-sensitive. It has improved my general health more than I dared imagine.'

*   *   *

'Selenium, after a month, has cured my nervous tension. I can cope a lot more with things.'

INDEX

ageing, process of, 10
American Ageing Association, 72
Andes, longevity in, 10
angina, 11
arthritis, 6, 24ff
   cure for, 23
   osteo, 27-8
   rheumatoid, 27-8
atherosclerosis, 63

blood pressure, high, 11
brewer's yeast, 11, 21
British Arthritic Association, 6,
   23, 24, 25, 31, 33

cancer, 10, 16, 21, 49, 50
   bladder, 60
   breast, 21, 49, 52, 54, 60
   colon, 53
   leukaemia, 54
   ovary, 53
   rectum, 54
   in sheep, 53
   stomach, 10, 49

Cancer and Its Nutritional Therapies,
   60
canning, 17
Crary, Dr E. J., 29
cystic fibrosis, 81

deoxyribonucleic acid (DNA), 51

Ecuador, longevity in, 38, 41
enzyme systems, 29
exercise, 13

film stars, 10
fish, 11
food additives, 17
free radicals, 51, 69
freezing, 17
Frost, Dr Douglas, 69, 76

garlic, 11, 21
goitre, causes of, 16

Harman, Dr Denman, 72
heart disease, 16, 21, 49

causes of, 64
heavy metal poisoning, 21
heredity, 10
Here's Health, 6, 23, 31, 33

journalists, 10

Keshan's disease, 61ff

Lancet, The 29
lawyers, 10

minerals, 13-6, 18
  chromium, 17
  copper, 17, 82
  iodine, 15-17
  iron, 15, 17
  magnesium, 17
  manganese, 28
  nickel, 20
  tin, 20
  vanadium, 20
  zinc, 28, 82
muscular dystrophy, 71
mushrooms, 11, 21

Norfolk, longevity in, 9, 11, 44

over-cooking, 17

Pakistan, longevity in, 39
Passwater, Dr Richard, 46, 57, 67, 76, 83
Phillips, Dr Roland, 42
preserving, 17
processed food, 14

rheumatism, 6
Robertson, Jean, 73
Russia, longevity in, 39

Schwartz, Klaus, 19
Schrauzer, Dr Gerard N., 52, 55, 56, 77
selenium, 11, 12, 17, 18, 19
  ACE, 24
  anti-inflammatory properties of, 25, 30
  deficiency, 61-3
  foods containing, 21, 74
  high level areas, 37
  low level areas, 19, 21, 75, 76
  supplements, 79
selenocystine, 59
sesame seeds, 11, 21
Shamberger, Dr, 77
shell-fish, 11
sodium selenite, 63
stress, 10

Thorn, Janet, 73
trace elements, 11, 13, 14, 16, 21
  areas with deficiencies, 16

ubiquinone, 67, 71
ulcers, 10

vitamins, 13, 14
  A, 15, 28, 51
  B-complex, 15
  C, 15, 28, 47, 51
  D, 15
  E, 15, 20, 21, 23, 26, 28, 46, 47, 51, 68ff, 82
  K, 15

wholegrain wheat, 11, 21
World Health Organization (WHO), 20, 65, 88, 89